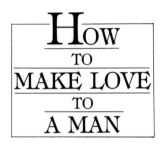

How
TO
MAKE LOVE
TO
A MAN

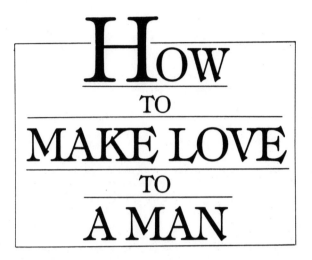

How
TO
MAKE LOVE
TO
A MAN

BY
ALEXANDRA PENNEY

SPECIAL CONSULTANT:
NORMAN F. STEVENS, JR.

WINGS BOOKS
NEW YORK • AVENEL, NEW JERSEY

The author gratefully acknowledges permission to reprint from the following:

Self, from an interview with Gay Talese by Sheila Weller, August 1980. By permission of *Self.*

Seduction Styles by Martha Pomroy and Martha Stilson-Caporale. © 1981 by M. Pomroy & M. Stilson-Caporale. By permission of the authors.

The Art of Eating by M.F.K. Fisher. Copyright 1949 by M.F.K. Fisher, renewed 1977 by Mary Kennedy Friede (M.F.K. Fisher). Reprinted with permission of Macmillan Publishing Company and Robert Lescher.

This 1986 edition is published by Wings Books, distributed by Outlet Book Company, Inc., a Random House Company, 40 Engelhard Avenue, Avenel, New Jersey 07001, by arrangement with Clarkson N. Potter, Inc.

Printed & Bound in the United States of America.

Library of Congress Cataloging-in-Publication Data

Penney, Alexandra.
    How to make love to a man.

    1. Sex instruction for women. 2. Men—Sexual behavior.
3. Sex (Psychology) I. Title
HQ29.P45   1986   613.9'6   85-17518
ISBN 0-517-60109-5

19 18 17 16

For Norman F. Stevens, Jr.

Acknowledgments

Without the intelligence, friendship and support of Charlotte Sheedy this book could never have happened. Grateful thanks also go to our friends and those who helped in many different ways who, for democratic reasons, are listed in alphabetical order: Dr. M. E. B., Myrna Blyth, Barbara Bonn, Edward Caracci, Jerry Chasen, Paul E. Cohen, Nancy de Sotto, Tuna B. Fish, Alice Fried, Asher Jason, Jeffrey Klomberg, Pamela Krausman, Anne Lederer, Harriet Love, Dr. T. M., David McCorkle, Phyllis Posnick, Susan Price, Martin Rapp, Alan Rosenberg, Leonard Russell, E. S., my talented editor Carol Southern, Suga, Larry Totah, Nancy Wechsler, my publisher Jane West, Phyllis Wilson and the waitresses at Coffee Connection.

Contents

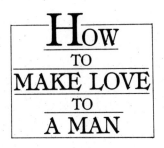

How
TO
MAKE LOVE
TO
A MAN

ONE

The Story of M.

No thanks," said the man on my right when our hostess offered him the most delicious dessert I had ever laid eyes on. As I began to attack the whipped cream with gusto (and guilt), I heard a barely audible groan.

"Oh, my God, just one bite," the man on my right pleaded, his fork twitching over my plate.

"*You* couldn't be on a diet. You can't *possibly* have weight problems. *You're* one of the blessed ones who were born tall and thin," I retorted, trying not to smile and protecting my pastry at all costs now that I had once again gone off my diet.

"Inside of me there's a screaming short fat person waiting to be let loose," he said with genuine seriousness. "*You* could never know the tortures I go through . . . the no-ice-cream cures, the whipped-cream withdrawals. . . ."

"You'll never know how much I understand *that*," I interrupted, liking him instantly for admitting his weaknesses.

"I'm a sweet freak too," I said, as I offered him the last succulent remnants from my dish.

We proceeded to finish two cups of black Sanka (no sugar), and for the next two hours we laughed and talked nonstop. I had just met him that evening and I was hoping now that he would ask to see me again. As we were about to say our good-byes and thank-yous, he said, "Would you like to come to my place for the rest of the evening?"

I tried to look sophisticated and worldly, as if this sort of thing was always happening to me at dinner parties. "I'd love to, but maybe we could meet for a dietetic lunch first?"

"Fine, what about this Thursday?"

"If I have anything else on my calendar, I'll break it," I said as suavely as I could possibly manage.

On Thursday I prepared for our lunch date with utmost care. I showered, fluffed on bath powder, used up a costly quantity of perfume (no cologne for *this* man), donned a pure silk slip that I saved for special occasions, abstained from breakfast, and in general tried to look as glamorous as the fates would allow.

When I entered the restaurant, the maître d' pointed out "Mr. Evans's table" and seated me.

"I've ordered you two peapods and a quail egg soufflé," announced Michael with a straight face as he poured champagne for me.

By the time we'd finished our second cup of espresso and split a sinful dessert, I had agreed to spend the coming weekend with him.

That evening, while I was having a long and knotty dialogue with myself about taking the risk of spending the weekend with a man I barely knew, Michael called to say he was especially looking forward to seeing me the next night at eight.

I washed my hair, treated it to an extra-penetrating conditioner, and began to look over some work I had brought home with me when I heard a scratchy noise coming from the letter slot downstairs. I pulled on a bathrobe, investigated, and found a pale gray envelope with my name handwritten on it. Inside was a single key and a short note:

Dear Joanna:

I hope to be home from the office tomorrow night by eight. In case I'm late, here is the key to my apartment. Please make yourself at home and comfortable.

M.

The key to his apartment! What kind of man gives you the key to his apartment unless you know him *very* well. I became a little uneasy. Even though he sounded liberated and we were soul mates in weight-watching, perhaps he was a closet macho type who intended me to cook his dinner (low-cal) and expected to find me ensconced in a negligee, his Old-fashioned in hand, when he walked in the door. Perhaps, let's face it — I let my imagination go all the way — perhaps he's kinky? I was a bit apprehensive but, more than that, I was curious. Michael was definitely intriguing and intelligent and romantic, and so, after more internal debating, I decided I'd keep the date.

At 8:05 the next evening I rang Michael's bell. No one answered. For God's sake, if this was such a romantic man, and if this was an evening he was so looking forward to, surely he could get away from his office before eight. I rang again. He may be a charmer, I thought, but he's definitely not considerate. My uneasiness was beginning to surface again. He has a responsible job and we were very properly introduced, an inner voice reminded me; go on, open the door, it said. I turned the key in the latch to face almost total darkness.

Two lone candles flickered, one with a note propped against it. He *is* kinky, I thought with a rising sense of panic. One foot wanted to fly out the door and the other wanted to walk — *very* cautiously — to where the note was. I advanced toward the small piece of paper which read:

BE DARING . . . COME IN

I heard a faint sound of music as my eyes became adjusted to the lack of light. If this is some kind of

joke . . . I thought. As I threaded my way toward the
strains of Roberta Flack I noticed that the whole
apartment was lit with small shimmering candles.
Following the path that the music set, I moved slowly
into the bedroom, where long-stemmed white roses
in a crystal vase shone through the dim light.

"Ah, you're here," said Michael, coming out of
what I took to be the bathroom. He was dressed in
jeans and a cream-colored cashmere sweater, looking
especially thin. "I'm glad to see," he continued, "that
you've got great homing instincts. Come, let's go
into the living room and have a drink."

By the time I finished my first glass of the iciest
champagne I had ever tasted, Michael and I were
laughing over my feelings of panic and my mood was
melting into one of total relaxation.

"Won't you take a bath?" he asked a while later.

"I've just had one!" I protested.

"Not like this," he said, leading me by the hand
into the bathroom, where he began running a bath,
adding rose petals and foamy azure-blue liquid to
the water.

"You look like an alchemist," I said.

He left the room, changed into a soft robe, and
sat beside me as I got into the scented blue water.
Next to me, on a small table with a single rose in a
simple vase, was a tray with white mushroom caps
filled with dark glistening caviar ("57 calories per,"

said a card on the plate). Michael fed me more champagne and slipped into the water with me. And later, in the cleanest, softest, whitest sheets, with the white roses giving off the most beautiful fragrance in the world, he made heavenly love to me.

•

The story of Michael was told to me by my closest friend, Joanna, and every word of it was true. "That night was the first time a man had ever made love to me," she said. "I had been to bed with men before, but Michael was the first man who truly made love to *me*, focused on *me*, made *my* fantasies come true, made love to me totally, imaginatively, perfectly."

But that wasn't the end! After that outrageously wonderful weekend, as Joanna began to know him better she began to realize that Michael wanted her to make love to him, too! A few weeks later he told her straight out, "Tomorrow night we have a special date to make love. Now it's up to *you*!"

This was the first time Joanna had ever heard a man, in or out of bed, say that he wanted to be made love to, that he wanted her to take charge, that he did not want always to be the one to take the full responsibility. There was no question in her mind. "I accept the challenge!" she told him.

As for me, this story, mad and fantastic as it sounded, made a huge impression. This, I believed strongly, was a story that had a vitally important issue at its heart. I began to wonder if Michael was unique in his ideas about women taking the initiative in making love to men, and if indeed men *wanted* to be made love to, did women know *how*? I realized that most women never think of making love to a man. We are taught that we should be seductive, entrancing, good conversationalists, and good cooks, but when it comes right down to bed, most of us want to be taken by Prince Charming to the fabulous land of orgasms and ecstatic sexual delights. Deep down, a woman *expects* a man to make love to her and to take the initiative in the sexual area.

I had read *The Joy of Sex*, and it had given me some good, basic technical pointers. I reread it to see if I had missed anything. Then I went out and bought *The Sensuous Woman, The Sensuous Man, Sex Without Guilt,* and *Love Without Fear,* and they had some interesting ideas but were not nearly specific enough. I turned to *More Joy of Sex, The Joy of Oral Sex,* and, in desperation, *The Joy of Gay Sex* (surely this would yield some interesting information). Most everything (except for the latter) seemed to take for granted that the male was basically the initiator in sex, that he should be sensitive to a woman's needs, take a lot of time, and help a woman achieve an orgasm or even many orgasms if she needed them.

But what, specifically, did *men* need besides an erection and a good climax? What were the finer pleasures that men responded to? No book or person had ever clearly revealed to women what making love to a man was really all about.

After my spree with the books I went to the primary source: I started asking men what they wanted from their wives, lovers, and/or mistresses. I interviewed over two hundred men of all ages from many different economic and ethnic backgrounds. Almost every one of them loved the idea of being made love to.

Herb, a six-foot-two construction engineer, came close to summing up the majority opinion. "Once in a while I want to lie back and be taken care of, just be a sex object." Alan, a free-lance photographer, agreed. "Lots of women are good at being made love to. They really enjoy sex, and that's gratifying to a man. But I've only known one or two who had a knack for making the fireworks go off for me. They were the greatest."

Other researchers are beginning to confirm that men want to be made love to. For example, in *Beyond the Male Myth: What Women Want to Know About Men's Sexuality*, the most striking statistic shows that 75 percent of men today want more involvement by the woman before or during intercourse. They want a woman who shows her interest and enjoyment, who is an active participant, and who is not timid in bed. This is a new attitude compared with that of men of past generations who wanted only compliance from their women. Until recently a man might have found an active partner threatening, unladylike, or downright sluttish, but most men today feel they are entitled to a pleasant respite from constantly having to prove their prowess.

Even if a woman senses that she *should* be more active sexually, *how* does she go about it without being threatening or aggressive? No one has ever helped women find out what their husbands or lovers need and no one has taught women step-by-step how to make love to men, in clear, simple, and unembarrassing language. In the following pages I hope to fill the gap.

How much or how little sexual experience you have had is not important. There are many women — as well as many men — who are highly experienced sexually, but this does not automatically make them good lovers. Technique will be covered in this book because *you must be technically good*. Most women have never been made aware of the importance of technique. They assume that making love is a natural experience and they'll instinctively know what to do. This is only partially true. You *do* know what to do instinctively, but there is a lot to be learned about what a man likes and when, where, and how he likes it. Men feel that women are lacking in know-how in certain crucial areas, and they're often too shy or embarrassed to let their wives or lovers know. Think about how many women suffered in silence until men learned what women needed physically and emotionally.

Technique is important, but making love is really a matter of understanding what your husband or lover wants in a *total* way. This totality includes his physical, emotional, and mental needs. Rich, full, satisfying lovemaking is one of the bases for the kind of intimate, long-lasting relationship that most of us are looking for or have and want to sustain. This book is about how to achieve that special kind of lovemaking through knowing more about *him*, so that ultimately *both* of you can participate in a deep, rewarding, enduring experience.

TWO

What's the Big Difference Between Men and Women?

Women like romance and affection. So do men. Women want sensitive, imaginative lovers. So do men. Women like to be passive. So, sometimes, do men. Women often feel insecure. Men, too. But beyond biology, there seem to be deep differences between men and women when it comes to specific attitudes toward sex.

Having Sex and Making Love

I found, in talking to hundreds of men, that the one most striking difference in attitude is the distinction many men make between "having sex" and "making love." Sometimes men want to have sex and sometimes they want to make love, and often they themselves are not fully aware of this duality. For most women, on the other hand, no matter how temporary or casual the relationship, there is usually an element of affection or caring in sex.

The important point to remember is this: once you understand a man's point of view, you'll have a much clearer idea of what he wants and needs in bed.

When it comes to making love, men are very much like women. Affection and caring are paramount. Making love is not just a matter of reaching physical satisfaction. It also involves two people who are helping each other reach emotional and spiritual fulfillment. When you have made love there is a feeling of having given and having received. It doesn't even matter how and when and who had an orgasm first, because making love is not just a purely physical act. Having sex, however, *is*.

To most men, having sex is basically a matter of relieving their own sexual tensions, and what their partners do or don't do is almost beside the point. Having sex means the same thing as "getting laid," and for men it is almost invariably a totally physical experience. There is very little caring or mutual concern involved, and it is most often a one-dimensional, one-sided, self-oriented activity. (There are some women who also compartmentalize sexual activity into loving sex and casual, impersonal sex, but they seem to be a small minority.)

Having sex, as I would define it, is almost wholly a physical experience with sexual services purchased or performed — not a very appealing concept. *There is, however, one important exception.* Pure physical sex can be perfectly terrific if you are with someone you care for, because there is an element of mutual fun and pure physical excitement about it. My friends Ed and Sally are a good example. They're a close, loving, committed couple who have been married for nearly ten years and have two children. Ed says that their lovemaking is "usually loving, considerate, frequent, and totally mutual. But sometimes," he says, "the urge just strikes me. Maybe it's excess energy or because I had a hard day at the office, but it's pure sex I want — it has nothing to do with the way I feel about Sally. I just want to get in bed and screw. Even though she may not be interested at first, she usually ends up getting turned on by how much I want it." Says Sally, "The first couple of times it happened I resented it . . . but I began to realize what an exciting, free feeling it is to let your body take over. I just put my mind on hold and let the sensations happen."

Unfortunately, too few women allow themselves to understand and enjoy the purely physical aspects of sexuality, and thus many men end up seeking sexual satisfaction away from home.

Many men say that they want to have sex or make love more frequently than their wives or lovers do. The statistics (in *Beyond the Male Myth*) show that 70 percent of the men interviewed want sex ideally at least three times a week, and about 50 percent want more sex than they are getting. However, the authors go on to state that "spontaneity and variety are more important than

frequency and are actually quite likely to lead to
increased frequency as intercourse becomes more
pleasurable."

The Madonna/Whore Syndrome

Underlying the making love/having sex duality
is the madonna/whore syndrome. There's an old
saying that goes: "A man wants a woman to be a lady
in the living room and a whore in his bed." Today,
many men would not put it this frontally, but it's true
that the madonna/whore concept of women is still a
fairly common one, especially in men over the age of
thirty-five. It stems from deep psychological roots
having to do with a man's forbidden sexual thoughts
about his mother (the madonna figure) and his
acceptable sexual desires for women of easy
accessibility (whores and prostitutes). Most men
synthesize these feelings as they mature, but,
psychological analysis aside, many sophisticated and
intelligent men still like to feel that they have a
Brigitte Bardot in the bedroom and a Princess Grace
in the living room.

Most men aren't even consciously aware that
they have contradictory feelings about women's
sexuality, and many women, too, put aside the
confusion they feel coming from men. "I thought my
marriage was fine. My husband treated me like a
goddess until he got bored with his own abstraction.
Then he went off with a carhop," says a woman who

was confronted with male double-think. "I realized," she says in retrospect, "that I accepted the role that he assigned to me."

If your husband or lover has mixed emotions about women's sexuality, the best thing to do is to bring the problem out into the open. You may find that he'll be surprised, relieved, and grateful for the recognition of these feelings of duality. Also, make an effort not to fall into *his* way of seeing women. If he isn't allowing you to express any of your instinctive, healthy, lustful feelings (or vice versa), be aware that this is a symptom of the madonna/whore duality. *Talk* to him about the problem before your roles become rigid and you end up symbolizing an unreal madonna or the woman he won't take out in public. Hopefully, the ideas in this book will help to free both men and women from the easy typecasting that limits sexuality. Good sex, as a man I know says, is "a healthy blending of ecstasy and lust."

THREE

The Surprising Six: Men's Biggest Sexual Fears

Women are great worriers when it comes to sex. Will he think I'm too hippy? Do my breasts droop too much? Do I smell funny? Is my cellulite so bad that I don't dare appear on the beach ever again? Will I ever achieve the mysterious Big Multiple O? Am I as good in bed as his old girl friend?

Men have their insecurities, too, although many men feel it's unmanly to talk about their problems, worries, and fears. However, if you ask questions and listen carefully, you'll find that a man's sexual concerns are quite different from yours and may cause him even more anxiety.

Size

Freud may have thought that penis envy applied to women, but I, for one, think he had it the wrong way around. "I know it's not true," said one man, "but I'm like a lot of men. Even when we know better, we feel deep down that 'the bigger your cock, the more of a man you are.'" "At the gym," says a Chicago lawyer, "everyone always checks out everyone else. But you have to make sure that no one sees you or they'll think you're gay." Explains a friend's college-age son, "You check out other guys' dongs because you want to know what your competition is." "When we were eight," recalls still another man, "my best friend and I took a ruler and measured our pee-pees. Mine was bigger." He's now thirty-seven, but there's still a residue of pride in his voice.

These are the facts: though penises are different in their flaccid state, they become much more similar when erect. The *average* size of the erect penis is six inches.

You run a risk if you make a direct statement about a man's penis. It may make him feel uncomfortable because it means to him that you're really noticing size (and making comparisons), and no matter what the size, he may have feelings of inadequacy. The safest rule to follow is stick to the truth or say nothing at all. If you feel his penis is medium to smallish, it's best not to comment, "Oh, how big!" because he'll pick up your insincerity, but no man minds hearing that his penis is beautiful.

A few men worry that their penises are *too* big and fear they will hurt their partners. This is rarely the case, because almost all vaginas can expand to the necessary size.

Temporary Impotence

Fear of impotence is perhaps the most crippling fear that a man can face. "When you have to come up with a hard-on, it's a very visual thing, there's no way around it," observes a carpenter. No man, from the young adolescent who is panicked about "getting it up" at the crucial moment, to the senior citizen who is worried about precisely the same thing, is immune to this fear. "*No man can will an erection*," Masters and Johnson write (the italics are theirs). The greatest cause of impotence is *fear* of impotence. There are definite things that you and your partner can do to allay the fear of impotence and actual temporary impotence itself. These are covered in Chapters 8 and 13.

Keeping It Up

Closely linked to anxiety about impotence is the very common fear men have that they will be unable to perform sexually. "Not only do you have to get it up, you have to keep it up," points out one man. He may have no trouble getting it up, but for him sexual encounters may produce intense anxiety because he worries that he will be an inadequate lover or, worse still, that he may be rejected because he has sexual shortcomings.

Coming Too Soon

Another common fear that men have is of premature ejaculation. "I'm always afraid I'll come in

ten seconds and I know it will screw everything up.
And the thought is often a self-fulfilling prophecy.
Then I'm in agony about how frustrated my partner
is when it happens," says one man who beat the
problem by seeing a sex therapist and learning how
to control ejaculation. (Often, however, couples will
consult a therapist together. Premature ejaculation
can usually be dealt with in the short time it takes to
learn simple controlling techniques.)

"Am I Gay?"

Some men fear that they will wake up one
morning and discover that they are gay. Just because
they have a momentary fantasy or imagined desire
(or even have had a homosexual contact), they think
that they are irretrievable closet cases. It should be a
comfort to know that research has shown that all of
us have natural bisexual feelings to some degree and
these emphatically do not mean that homosexuality
is going to become a way of life.

Aging

Although most men are anxious about losing
their hair and developing a paunch, what they fear
most about aging is that they will no longer be able to
function in bed. It's true that men are at a sexual peak
at eighteen, but, as Kinsey showed, at age sixty the
average male has sex once a week. Since this is the
average man, it means that many men are having sex

more often at that age. In addition, recent studies show that a healthy man can be sexually active as long as he lives.

There are other fears that some men have, such as the fear of "wasting sperm" because it is a "life force," limited in amount, and can be depleted. Production of sperm *does* diminish with age but never disappears completely.

No one in this world is fear-free. If you're aware of the fears that most men have, you'll be able to cooperate in trying to alleviate or, better yet, eliminate them. Once you recognize that men aren't perfectly tuned sex machines — they're lovably human — and you become sensitive to their special problems, you've taken a giant step toward breaking down barriers that stand in the way of love and intimacy.

FOUR

Giving Yourself Permission

Women are too uptight.

For a lot of women sex is in the head. If women just followed their guts instead of thinking and thinking, they'd be much better off. Women like to call themselves sexy and wild in bed, but very few really are.

— Two anonymous men

This chapter is about liberation. It's about freeing and opening your own mind to pleasure so that you can pleasure a man completely. It's about abandoning yourself to passion without hearing voices from the past whispering to you that "good girls don't have those feelings, good girls don't do those things."

It stands to reason that a woman whose fears, prejudices, and inhibitions tell her "stop" at every step is not likely to get very far on the road to sexual fulfillment for herself or her partner. If you've been trained to believe that genitals are nasty, for instance, you'll have difficulty caressing your lover's penis in a way that gives you both pleasure, let alone using your mouth in creative, sensuous ways. If you've been programmed to see sex as a "marital duty," something to be done in the dark, with as little fuss as possible, how will you be able to achieve the kind of physical and emotional freedom that takes lovemaking out of the realm of everyday experience? A woman who has given herself permission to truly enjoy sex is the one who can give extraordinary pleasure to a man.

What's stopping you from enjoying your own healthy sexuality? Perhaps, like many of us, you've been subjected to a more or less subtle variety of "good girl" training. If you still feel uncomfortable picking up the phone and calling a man first, you may still believe, at some level, that you're supposed to sit back and let a man make all the moves. Not many brides are being counseled to "lie back and think of England" these days, but many of us, especially over a certain age, still can't allow ourselves to feel free or spontaneous or comfortable about our own sexuality. The outdated subliminal message still lingers in the recesses of our minds: nice girls don't enjoy sex.

On the other hand, women constantly see and hear conflicting and equally powerful messages.

Wherever you look, articles tell you how to enjoy sex more and more and more. Movies and television promote the idea that sex is the be-all and end-all of existence, and that bad girls are definitely having more fun. Psychiatrists and therapists will tell you that it's necessary to enjoy sexuality and participate in it wholeheartedly to achieve mental and physical well-being. No wonder many women find themselves in a difficult double bind. As a magazine researcher complained, "We grew up hearing one thing about sex, and now we're told something completely different. It's not surprising that a grown-up intelligent woman can be confused, if not paralyzed, when she gets into bed with a man."

If you can identify with this double bind in yourself, one of the ways out is to take sex one small step at a time. First, start reading as much as you can about the subject. Having concrete, specific information about what to do, how to do it, and when to do it will help defuse your anxieties. If you feel that your inhibitions are seriously affecting your relationship with your husband or lover, don't hesitate to talk to a therapist or sex counselor. In many cases, just a few sessions can clarify your problem areas and help you change your attitudes. The chapters that follow should also help you demystify sex and alleviate your anxieties. You'll see, by all your reading and research, that nothing in sex (unless it is harmful to you or to someone else) is *bad*. Armed with reassurance and information, you should be able to begin to deal with the realities of the bedroom in a much more relaxed way.

Do *only* the things you feel comfortable with, and then, very cautiously, begin to explore more and more areas, remembering that if you take small steps you're less likely to feel overwhelmed and nervous. If your husband or lover asks or implies that he would like to try something that you're not ready for, tell him honestly you're not there — *yet*. If you've been thoroughly programmed with the "good girls don't do *that*" idea, don't expect to shed your inhibitions and become a lusty, free-thinking woman overnight. It may also comfort you to know that a great many women (and many men too) have problems with letting go and feeling free about their sexuality. Unresolved emotions can put the brakes on your sexual motivation, too. If you're angry with your mate and haven't resolved those negative, hostile feelings, it is almost impossible to keep an open receptive attitude toward sexuality.

Making love also means allowing yourself to take the risk of becoming involved with another person in the most intimate and complex way, and allowing that other person to know you totally. Making love is an intimate act which, when repeated with the same partner over a period of time, can unfold and reveal new and deeper levels in each, thus creating the closest and most meaningful kind of bond.

To become intimate with someone also involves the fear of exposing the most private parts of you.

Fear is actually the biggest obstacle to sexual pleasure: the fear of being hurt physically or emotionally, the fear of approaching someone, the fear of being rejected, the fear of making a mistake, the fear of being ridiculous, undesirable, incompetent, clumsy, foolish, ugly, insensitive — to name but a few. Realize that *both* of you have fears and *both* of you are vulnerable. As one man astutely observed, "For sex to be everything it can be, you can't just stand physically naked. You have to undress emotionally too, and there is a great deal of vulnerability involved. If you are able to take the risk emotionally and physically, you're leaving yourself open for high-quality sex."

FIVE

On Aggressiveness

As a partner in a conservative brokerage firm in Houston, Stewart is a man who is accustomed to directing hundreds of people and manipulating millions of dollars daily. A tall, attractive athletic-looking widower of fifty-two, he is one of the most eligible men in Texas. He's also honorary chairman of one of Houston's major fund-raising drives. On a Tuesday morning several months ago he found himself in his mahogany-paneled office face to face with a reporter from one of the city's daily newspapers.

"She asked me about the current fund drive, about the projected figures, about the percentage of administrative costs for the charity, about the pictures of my children on my desk, about what I was doing for dinner that evening. I had never been approached so directly by a woman, and I was charmed — Nina made all the plans, led me like a lamb to her favorite small neighborhood restaurant. She even suggested a wine. I'd never met a woman who dared to do that with me. When I asked for the check, the waiter said to me, 'Everything's been taken care of, sir.' I found out later that Nina had arranged to have the bill sent to her."

"Stewart was so involved in business he hardly noticed that I was a woman," explains Nina. "But I thought he was a very interesting man. Power is sexy, you know. . . . But the real reason we get along so well is we both know how to make things happen. Our relationship would never have developed if I hadn't made the first move."

Among their most recent moves have been a romantic two days at his hideaway in the mountains, and another equally romantic two days spent painting Nina's kitchen.

"Nina is as decisive and aggressive about what she wants in bed as she is about everything else," says Stewart. "For a man like me it's a new and exciting experience to just lie back and have a woman take care of things."

After I'd been doing interviews on the subject of sex for several months, I realized that, over and over again, one phrase — "aggressive woman" — provoked supercharged emotional responses, particularly from women. A surprising number of women feel deeply that if they take the initiative and let a husband or lover know what they want, they're sure to be seen as threatening, unfeminine, aggressive, pushy, a turnoff. Gay Talese, the man who did nine years of research before writing *Thy Neighbor's Wife*, disagrees. In an interview in *Self* magazine he states:

Men need help. A lot of them are passive. I think most men would welcome more sexually aggressive women. A woman who's uninhibited about taking charge of her own sexual pleasure – and his – whether by making the initial approach socially or being assertive in the sex act itself – is a boon to a man, not a threat.

Furthermore, he adds:

Many women feel that a man will be threatened if they are assertive or make the first move sexually. If she's subtle and intelligent about it, no man should ever feel threatened. If he does, he is a man who's more comfortable putting the blame on women instead of where it belongs: on himself.

Almost all the men I spoke with agree with Mr. Talese. A well-known, highly experienced film producer claims, "I like an aggressive woman. To me, aggressiveness means self-assurance, action, a lack of passivity, a forward kind of thinking, and that's a definite plus. Where I think that things get into trouble is when a woman tries to become the dominating figure in a relationship. She can be dominant some of the time, but there's got to be a healthy balance."

An executive at a midwestern retail chain who has been joyfully married for eight years to, as he put it, "a woman that most people would call profoundly aggressive," defined an aggressive female as "any woman who has a sense of her self and, you know, that's a positive attribute." The word "aggressive," as it pertains to women, he suggests, is used by men for the wrong reasons. "It's basically not the idea of an aggressive woman that scares men to death; it's the woman who will not play a traditional role of passivity. The word 'aggressive' today is a catchword, and it is hiding the basic fright of dealing with a woman who is an equal partner."

Exactly how do you go about letting a man know what you want and try to give him what you suspect *he* wants without being negatively aggressive, or acting "pushy"? You do it by using intelligence, sensitivity, subtlety, and femininity. This emphatically means that you do *not* pretend, tease, manipulate, submit, or play any roles. You are the essence of *female*, the essence of *yourself*, because, ultimately, the male's physiological and psychological response is dependent on femaleness. He can't be ready for lovemaking unless he is stimulated by a female presence. One man said it this way: "I want to go to bed with a feminine woman, and she can be aggressive. There's a way of being aggressive — a *female* kind of aggressive. It's really a new way of stating that a modern woman can be seductive — and it's wonderful. There's a kind of male aggressive which is tough and dominating, and which can also be interesting, but if that was what I was looking for, I'd go to bed with a man."

Men say that one of the best ways a woman can indicate she's interested is to *look at a man directly*. This may seem like a simple gesture, but for many women it is extremely difficult to do. Many women shy away from direct eye contact with a man because they feel there's something brazen about it. Many a man feels that a woman who looks his way — and *holds* the look — is making an initial contact in a very seductive way. There's another term for this kind of direct look: bedroom eyes. "A woman who catches my eye is saying, 'I'd like to get to know you better,'" states one man. "If I'm interested I can easily find some excuse to talk to her, or ask her for a drink, and if I'm not interested, I just look in the other direction. No one is hurt, no one feels rejected."

When it comes to eye contact, men note that if you look at them directly, you're paying a compliment, especially if you add a smile. If you look in a man's eyes and then zero in on the crotch, that's going too far. It's not seductive; it's just plain vulgar.

Another way to show you're interested is simply by *talking to him*. One clever woman I talked with suggested using a trick that film femmes fatales do: keep your hands and body completely still and focus in on him with your eyes. You don't have to wait until he talks to you first. Start up a conversation related directly to the situation at hand. *Don't* talk about yourself. Ask him what he thinks of that painting in the corner, or the hors d'oeuvres that are being served, or tell him you like the cologne he's wearing, what's the name of it? Another sexy woman believes that talking about work when you've just met someone can send him flying in the other direction. "Ask him who cut his hair," she advises. "It's safer."

Another approach men say can be seductive is to use old cliché opening lines that can humorously lead the way to further conversation. "May I offer you a light?" is what a man usually says to a woman. Turn the tables and try it out on him. Other old standbys that have worked are: "I'd love to buy you a cup of coffee" or "Can I buy you a drink?" Just remember to keep the comment appropriate to the occasion. "I once found myself at a dreadful cocktail party in a tacky motel bar," a woman executive told me. "In desperation, I turned to the only interesting-looking man in the room and asked, 'What's a nice guy like you doing in a place like this?' Four years later, we're still friends."

One other trick to letting a man know he is the object of your interest is to put yourself in close physical proximity to him — *gently* invade his space. A seductive woman describes this approach at a party: "Just keep putting yourself near him and all the while keep concentrating on something else, a person, a painting, a shelf of books. Finally you work it so that you're sitting next to him or standing by him and you're just a shade too close. You are directly invading his personal territory. You know how pigeons are all perfectly spaced when you see them perched on telephone wires? If one moves, then the whole pattern is upset? *You* are the one who's upsetting the pattern to get his attention. He'll feel it, and if he's interested, he'll respond."

A more daring, more imaginative way of suggesting to a man that you'd be delighted at the idea of knowing him better is to send him something. Flowers or a plant can often be the perfect way to say what you find difficult to express verbally. A magazine editor who felt uneasy about calling a man directly, sent a single long-stemmed Gloriana lily with a card inviting the doctor she'd recently met to dinner. He found the gesture very seductive. "This was the first time a woman had sent me flowers, or rather, a flower, and I liked it very much. It made me think, she's unusual, she does the unexpected. It was the perfect touch."

Whatever you send, it should show imagination and be *personal*. Freshly baked muffins or banana bread dropped off at his office in time for the midmorning coffee break, specially ground and blended coffee for a coffee lover, a late-night special delivery of ice cream for a sweet freak, a poster from an art exhibition for an art lover, homemade linguine for the pasta lover: the list of ideas is endless. *What* you send, and *how* you send it (mail, messenger, UPS, local boy or girl scout, even carrier pigeon), shows what kind of person *you* are and that you've taken the time to think about what kind of man *he* is. These are the kinds of gestures that aren't aggressive, they're endearing.

Men are very definite in their opinions about what is anti-seductive. Gestures and attitudes that are too crude, too obvious, too insensitive, produce a highly negative effect that men label aggressive and pushy. The men I polled say that the following are major turnoffs for them:

The pressure cooker.

This is the woman who is constantly putting pressure on a man. She does *all* the calling and *all* the pursuing. What's left for him to do? Find another woman who will let *him* be responsible, at least in part, for the relationship. A relationship involves *two* people both working to make something happen between them, right from the beginning.

The crotch-grabber.

She's the kind of woman men find most unappealing. "I don't know what's happening with some women, but I find I'm assaulted, right on the crotch. Maybe it's Women's Lib and they think they should be very direct. I don't like it. Why doesn't she just slip her hand in my pocket instead, if she's going in that direction?" asked one man. Another suggested, "I don't want my girl friend to treat me like a sex object. Just a feathery gesture at first and then maybe another light touch so that I'm pretty clear on what her motives are — that's okay with me — but I don't want her to go straight to the point so fast!"

The draper.

This is the woman who drapes herself in public over a man's neck, shoulders, wherever. "Even if I were very turned on to a woman and she came over to me and hung on me in a suggestive way when there were other people present, I don't think I could respond. It's just not a pretty way to act," stated one man.

The lap-sitter.

She is closely related to the draper. "Any woman who comes and sits on my lap at a party embarrasses me," claims one man, and many others agree. "Maybe it's because I'm afraid I'll get a hard-on, but more probably it's because I think a woman's being too pushy. It's a different story if we're just home alone and the girl I'm involved with makes herself cozy in my lap. I love that," he says.

The pushy kisser.

Kissing can be affectionate, friendly, romantic, sensual, erotic. A kiss is a meeting of two pairs of lips. If one of those pairs is overly insistent, *that's* a pushy kisser.

The tentative woman.

She's the one who comes across as lacking self-assurance and self-confidence. "Tell women not to be tentative or timid about what they're doing or what they're touching or what they're saying when they're with a man. It makes a man feel that a woman is ambivalent about what she's doing and that maybe she feels she shouldn't be there because she's doing something bad," advises one bachelor. "A woman who isn't clear about the fact that she's doing the right thing transmits that uneasy feeling to her partner, and it's usually the opposite of what she's hoping to achieve," says another.

The bad-timer.

There's one last trait too often found among women that is completely counterseductive and seems to be a universal problem for men: it's the lack of a sense of timing. No matter what your approach, it will never work if you're insensitive to your man's needs at the moment. You may be as subtle and romantic and provocative as any man could wish, but when he's off to a football game or a workout at the gym or an appointment with a car salesman, if he's like most of his sex, he won't be interested — he has other things on his mind. Put yourself in his place. If you were going out to a museum or shopping with your best friend, would you cancel out if your man wanted to make love to you? You might — or you might not, but that seems to be one of the interesting differences between men and women!

SIX

Getting Ready: Feeling Sexy

If you ask one hundred men, "What is sexy?"
ninety-nine of them will probably say something
like "self-confidence" or "self-assurance." The other
one will always say "big boobs." I don't think those
ninety-nine are lying. They really don't care that
much if a woman is beautiful or has a goddesslike
form. What they really think is sexy is the woman
who is confident and feels good about herself and her
body.

It's amazing how many of us *don't* feel attractive
or desirable or comfortable with our bodies. Susan, a
genuinely pretty thirty-one-year-old executive
secretary who has a mop of auburn curls and the kind
of poreless porcelain skin that most of us dream
about, says, "I can feel sexy with my clothes on. But
the minute I take them off I become very conscious of
my broad backside. I spend too much time and
energy trying to hide it from my lover."

Many women feel the same way. They prefer to keep the lights down low or turned off altogether when they make love. Others are hesitant to try out new positions because they think they'll be displaying too much flesh and too little muscle tone. In short, many women don't think they're sexy.

It's worth reviewing the words men use most often when they try to define "sexy":

self-confidence	clean
composure	neat
intelligence	well-groomed
self-assurance	healthy
friendliness	attractive
femininity	real
at ease with her body	fit

So, contrary to what the media say, you do *not* have to be beautiful or to have a perfect body to be truly sexy. Many of our insecurities and our fears are amplified when we watch TV or go to the movies, or leaf through glossy fashion magazines telling us that people with beautiful faces and beautiful bodies are the ones who are sexy and have all the fun. "If you *feel* that you are sexy, men will feel that you are too," states a present-day courtesan, and at least three terrific men I know think *she's* the sexiest creature on earth. This is a woman who moves as if she had a great body, even though her hips are more than generous and her legs would never stop traffic.

What does it take to feel sexy? Simply this: the more you are comfortable and at ease with yourself and your body, the more sexy and attractive you will feel, and *you must feel sexy in order to be sexy*.

Very, very, very few people have super bodies and/or flawless faces, and it's important to keep this thought in mind. If you don't, you're likely to fall into some very common traps that you can set for yourself about how you look: the "either I look terrific or I look terrible" trap, the "he's going to notice my blemishes" trap, and the "constant comparison" trap. There will *always* be a body or a face better than yours, so if you see yourself in these negative terms, you're inevitably going to assume that there's something not right about you, and you'll constantly feel inadequate and unattractive.

Suppose, now you know the traps, you still aren't pleased with yourself. The best, quickest, and most efficient course of action is to start a serious diet and/or exercise program. The minute you begin, the process of feeling more self-assured — and more sexy — has begun.

Once you're launched on an exercise program, it's time to look critically at some other areas. Is your makeup becoming, or have you gotten stuck in a time warp as some women do? These are women who have stayed with outdated looks such as painted doe eyes or chocolate-brown lipstick. The same goes for your hair: is it styled in a contemporary way? Does it look clean and healthy? Are your hands and feet cared for? Over and over again, men from every social and economic background say that they check out details such as makeup, hair, nails, and skin. They don't need to be with a stunning woman, but they definitely do prefer women who take time to make themselves look their best. One man sums it up by stating, "I look for the details, the things that show the kind of woman she is. If she's careful about herself and her body, I think that's a big factor in being a sexy woman." Pampering and caring for yourself is not self-indulgence. It can make you feel sexy, and if you *feel* sexy and delicious, you'll transmit that message.

There's one more thing you can do to get your message across in a very specific way: start right now to practice some pelvic exercises. If you can control your pelvic movements you're going to feel — and be — more sexy.

Pelvic Control: the Sexy Woman's Secret

As one man whose discerning eye covers Manhattan's famous discotheques sums up, "You can usually tell if a woman really knows how to make love from the way she moves when she dances. She moves her fanny in the sexiest way and she swivels her hips while her shoulders stay straight. When I spot one of those I know she's a killer. And I've never been wrong when I've been able to get to know that woman."

You don't have to be a disco queen to move your pelvis in the right way. You can learn to make the movements with concentration and work. A leading exercise studio for women here in New York has a knowledgeable director who believes totally in the necessity of pelvic control, not only for the well-being of the total body but for the well-being of sexual relationships. Her classes heavily emphasize pelvic tilts, rotation of the pelvis (a movement very much like a "bump and grind"), and muscle control, all of which give ease and freedom of movement to the lower half of the body. Take some time each day to practice pelvic exercises; the results, as your man will be sure to tell you, will be well worth the effort.

The first exercise in pelvic control is aimed at tightening and relaxing the interior muscles surrounding the vagina in order to give more intense sensations to your partner. Specifically, he'll feel heightened pleasure when his penis is in direct contact with firm vaginal walls that seem to clasp and unclasp it.

In order to isolate the muscle that you need to tighten and relax, sit on the toilet and spread your legs wide apart. As you urinate, try starting and stopping the flow. The muscle that you are using is your target. Once your have located this muscle, practice tightening and relaxing it every day. Repeat the movement at least 40 to 50 times per day to get the muscle in top shape. This is a "secret" exercise that you can do almost anywhere and no one will be the wiser (except your lover), so practice it at home, at your desk, in elevators, on buses, wherever. After a month or so, you can drop the repetitions to 20 times a day to maintain elasticity of the muscle — not counting the times you are exercising while you make love.

The second step to pelvic control involves doing two basic exercises that concentrate on the lifting and rotation of the pelvis. The dance floor is not the only place where you can use these kinds of movements. You should know how to move your pelvis when you are making love to give you greater contact and friction with your partner in the genital area, thus heightening the range of sensations you are both feeling.

The best way to learn a pelvic tilt is to imagine that you are putting on the tightest pair of jeans you can fit yourself into. Standing with your legs about twelve inches apart, your knees bent, imagine that you have pulled up the pants and you are now going to zip up the zipper. As you do your imaginary zip, your pelvis should be tilted forward, your stomach held in tightly, and your seat tucked under. Once you are in that position, hold it for a second, and then let go, then repeat the zipping, thrusting-forward movement once again. Your knees and feet should stay in place; only your pelvis should be tilting backward and forward, about three to four inches at most. Repeat this movement about 20 times a day until you can do it without thinking about it. This should take anywhere from one to four days. When you have mastered this, it's time to add a rotating movement to the tilt.

The rotating movement is similar to the bump and grind that you've seen dancers do. Belly dancers are especially adept at this one. Many women have gone to belly-dancing classes at their local "Y" specifically to perfect their pelvic control as well as to learn to move in a sinuous and sexy way.

The first step in pelvic rotation is to stand with your feet about twelve inches apart, knees slightly bent, fanny tucked under, arms at your sides, body relaxed. Very slowly tilt your pelvis forward (as you did in the simple pelvic tilt) and then far to the right, putting most of your weight on your right foot. Now tilt your pelvis to the back (your fanny is pushed back and up) and then rotate your pelvis to the left, putting your weight on your left foot. Next tilt your pelvis forward and tuck your fanny under while rotating over to the right foot again, thus completing one circular movement. This can be a tricky set of motions to master, so do them very slowly at first, consciously thinking out each movement. After you have done 10 rotations, reverse your movements and rotate your pelvis in the opposite direction. Repeat the rotation 10 times in each direction until you are moving easily and smoothly. Some women say it helps a great deal to practice to music.

Once you have become skilled in the pelvic tilt plus rotation, you're ready for the expert's category by combining these movements with your interior tightening and relaxing movements. The combination of these two gives you almost perfect pelvic control while you are making love, thus allowing you to give your partner and yourself a whole new range of physical sensations that heighten both his and your pleasure immeasurably.

Begin by standing, as for pelvic rotation, with

your feet about twelve inches apart, knees slightly bent, fanny tucked under, pelvis forward. With your pelvis in this position, make your interior tightening movement. Now lean to the right and relax the interior muscle. Tilt and rotate to the back, fanny pushed up, tightening again, then to the left, relaxing the interior muscle. Do this to the count of 4:

1. Forward tilt — tighten.
2. Right — relax.
3. Back tilt — tighten.
4. Left — relax.

What you're aiming for is a combination of a tightening and relaxing of the interior muscles while you are tilting and rotating. At first the two motions can seem as difficult as rubbing your head and patting your tummy at the same time, but if you do them very slowly and count each movement out loud, you'll find that you will soon be able to do the two motions simultaneously. Start out by doing 20 tilt/tighten rotations a day, and work up to 40 by the end of two weeks. At the end of two weeks the two motions should be coming together naturally without your thinking about them. After you've mastered the movements, you don't need to keep practicing. You'll actually begin to use them when you make love. (How you'll use them, and what for, is discussed fully in Chapter 11.)

By the way, one woman who told her husband that she was "seriously practicing pelvic control" discovered that not only was he amused, he was aroused.

SEVEN

Setting the Scene

G reece had its hetaerae, Rome its delicatae, and Japan has its geishas, but perhaps the most famous women who left a legacy of seduction and lovemaking with elaborate, lavish preparations, were the nineteenth-century women of France, known as courtesans or *les grandes horizontales*.

The great French courtesans were highly regarded by most members of society even though they were paid for their work — making love. It is notable that many of the great courtesans were not beautiful or even pretty, but they were extraordinarily and uniquely educated in their ability to heighten a man's pleasure, and thus they were paid extravagantly, not only with money, but with houses, jewels, and servants. They, in turn, spent extravagant sums to please their lovers.

Courtesans of the last century thought nothing of ordering vanloads of rare orchids to be strewn on the parquet floors of their châteaux so that their lovers could feel the exquisite sensation of crushing the soft blossoms with their feet. They spent a great deal of time and effort arranging for delicacies of every sort for their lovers, and champagne, the "wine of love," flowed without end. One courtesan, known especially for her wit and wild antics, promised her lover and her guests that she would give them meat too tender to be cut, whereupon she disappeared. A few minutes later, naked, draped with parsley and emeralds to match, she was carried into the dining hall on a silver salver by four strapping costumed manservants, torsos bared, with color-coordinated jewels in their navels.

Another courtesan ordered a solid silver double-sized bathtub with lapis and jade faucets so that she could bathe sensuously with her admirers. Silk and satin sheets were the rule; each time a lover was expected, the sheets were changed so that his crest or monogram would be immediately visible and he would feel comfortable and at home. Perfumes in crystal and silver jars, particularly ambergris, thought to be an aphrodisiac, were sprayed by special servants throughout the perfectly appointed rooms.

One courtesan always sent *toilettes de nuit*, two or three dozen nightgowns and peignoirs in different colors, to her various lovers, so that each could choose his favorite color for their night of love. Another had her dog dyed a special shade of blue, the preferred hue of her current duke.

Underlying all this extravagance was a very specific intention. The courtesan wanted to stimulate and please her lover. In particular, she wanted to focus on the pleasures of the senses. Thus flowers were arranged in his favorite colors to please his eye, food was chosen to satisfy his particular palate, fragrance was used to enchant his sense of smell, his favorite music was to be heard at dinner and in the bedroom, sheets and pillows accentuated the pleasure of touch. The courtesan was also keenly aware of the art of lively and interesting conversation. Thus she developed not only the art of pleasuring the senses but her own sense of wit and humor, as well as making herself familiar with her lover's business and the news of the day.

•

The great French courtesans were a phenomenon of the nineteenth century, and their showiness was a result of the enormous sums they were paid for making love in the most complete way, but underneath all their extravagance was a genuine concern for giving sensual and sexual pleasure to men. To me, courtesans are fascinating women who were the ultimate practitioners in pleasing a man's senses while making him feel completely at home. In other words, they knew how to seduce and how to set the scene for lovemaking. If you take the time to think about what your husband or lover responds to, and if you remember to pleasure *each* of his senses, you will have discovered the courtesans' greatest secret. The important point is to set, not a scene that pleases *you*, but one that delights and inspires your particular man. Here are some ideas you can use as take-off points.

Sense of sound.

"Music," says a Los Angeles architect, "can be a powerful aphrodisiac. Certain slow, driving beats — the classic is Ravel's *Bolero* — have a definite sexual rhythm. Ricky Lee Jones and Donna Summer, although they are opposites, can have the same turn-on effect." Choose records or tapes that *he* will respond to; if he's involved with New Wave, playing country and western is more than likely an inappropriate gesture. Some men are soothed by the sounds of a Mozart sonata and feel like crawling undercover when they hear rock or disco beats, while others like their music gutsy and booming. It doesn't take long to find out what he's tuned into.

Perhaps, however, his sense of sound has been bombarded all day with telephones, typewriters, honking horns, and screaming sirens. In this case you might be pleasuring him by blocking out all noise, turning off the telephone and TV, and giving his ears a well-earned rest.

Many people have special records that set the mood for romance or become a signal that means making love. "I asked Michael to make a list of the ten records he thought were the most romantic ever," my friend Joanna told me. "Number one was Edith Piaf's album that had 'La Vie en Rose' on it, next was 'The Impressionists,' after that was a Roberta Flack album, a Neil Diamond one, and then came *Tosca*."

Sense of sight.

We've all seen men watch women as they walk down the street. Notice how men also linger over a provocative picture in a magazine or how some males almost automatically check out a woman's chest area. Men's responses vary widely, but in general most men quickly react to visual stimuli. You can easily set some interesting and provocative scenes for him at home: a bed turned down the way it is in a hotel, a specially set table with candles and flowers, you in a steamy bubble bath when he comes home, sheer black stockings draped over a bedroom chair, a book of erotic pictures placed in a conspicuous spot. "Every man I know," says Sheila, a very seductive executive secretary, "is turned on by a book of photographs by Helmut Newton. It's called *White Women*. I keep it right on the coffee table."

Keep in mind, however, that what stimulates one man could cause embarrassment to another; size up his particular likes and dislikes or get to know his preferences and please him accordingly.

How he sees the bedroom is another interesting point. Martha Pomroy and Martha Stilson–Caporale, two writers who did an informal survey on men's preferences about bedrooms, say that "the seductive bedroom, from a man's point of view, would never appear in *Playboy* magazine." These were the results of their survey on the ideal bedroom: the preferred color is blue; wall-to-wall ranks way above any kind of shag carpeting; the bed is queen-size or larger, with an inner-spring mattress (foam is too hot in the summer); four or more pillows are the "correct" number; bedside tables should be free from clutter; television and radio are important props; and lots of plants are essential. The composite picture of the seductive bedroom, then, according to their informants, is one that reflects nature. "When making love," the authors conclude, "men were on a grassy hilltop under a blue sky surrounded by lush vegetation!"

Sense of smell.

Most men are not as aware as women are of the power of fragrance and its aphrodisiac effects. Give him a bath with some scented bath oil, place a fragrant soap at the sink, spray your sheets and pillows very lightly with the fragrance that you use. Dab some of your personal perfume on the light bulbs; when the bulbs are turned on, the heat will diffuse the fragrance in the room. Fragrance is a very powerful subliminal signal that makes a man aware of your presence, but use it with restraint. Too much perfume sprayed on you, your clothes, the sheets, the room, can be overpowering and send him running out the door in search of fresh air.

Sense of touch.

Men claim that things that feel silky or are diaphanous are very feminine and therefore *very sexy*. That explains why so many of them respond to silky, see-through nightgowns and underwear and soft sheets that feel smooth and satiny. Fragile glasses and delicate plates and cups also have a feminine feeling about them that men find seductive to the touch. They say it makes them more aware of their own masculinity. Shiny, clean, healthy-looking hair is something else men say they love to feel. And almost every man agrees that a soft, clingy dress made from flowing material is something that almost asks to be touched. Ditto for silky nightgowns, robes, and underwear. It's also quite surprising to find out how many men have a secret passion to touch a pair of pure silk bikini underpants. "Silk," says a sensuous friend of mine, "holds your scent better than nylon."

Sense of taste.

The old cliché goes, "the quickest way to a man's heart is through his stomach." It's true — and rarely does a man deny it. To prepare a meal for someone is one of the most loving and seductive gestures a woman can make. Historically, breaking bread or the sharing of food is the beginning of closeness between people.

The great gastronomer M. F. K. Fisher writes wonderfully about foods for seduction. The great courtesans, she says, studied the appetites of their prey.

. . . Once caught, the human male is studied by the huntress as thoroughly as if he were a diamond. . . . She analyzes his motor reflexes after he has downed a fair portion of jugged venison, and if instead of showing a pleasurable skittishness he yawns and puffs and blinks, she nevermore serves that gamy dish. She notes coldly, calculatingly, his reactions to wine and ale and heady spirits, as well as to fruits, eggs, cucumbers and such; she learns his dietetic tolerance, in short, and his rate of metabolism, and his tendencies toward gastric as well as emotional indigestion. And all this happens whether she be a

*designing farm girl in Arkansas or a slim worldly
beauty on the Cap d'Antibes.*

Every man's sense of taste is highly individual.
Some men have highly refined palates and will
appreciate the time and effort that go into making a
gourmet meal. Others will respond to the
thoughtfulness of a woman who prepares their
favorite dish, even if it's only a plain (but juicy)
hamburger or a specially selected TV dinner to be
enjoyed with their preferred brand of beer.

An imaginative man once suggested to a friend
of mine that she plan a wine-tasting session *à deux*
consisting of half bottles of wines from different
countries. If your man is not a drinker — or if he's on
a diet — try an exotic-sounding mineral water. A
chilled bottle of sparkling water is a special,
inexpensive (and no-calorie) drink to have before or
during dinner.

The point to remember about taste is that it's *his*
taste you're trying to captivate. Don't give him what
you *think* he likes: take the time to find out his
special preferences. "I eat out at restaurants so
much," says a sophisticated single New York man,
"I'm the guy who appreciates a plain old homey meat
loaf instead of a fancy dinner." *You* might find
hamburger or meat loaf just Too Boring, but if you fix
it for him it may endear you to him forever!

EIGHT

Beating the Jitters

There's something wonderfully exciting about the prospect of going to bed with someone for the first time. But although you may be looking forward to it, you're likely to feel uneasy about it, too. One friend of mine says candidly, "I'm a little afraid. I hope it's going to be great, but I'm worried that it's going to be awkward, that I'm not going to look good to him, and that things won't be as perfect as I want them to be." The first time is *rarely ever* perfect. Bodies are bared, emotions are flying, and anxiety is peaking. There's *always* a natural awkwardness about having a sexual experience with someone new, particularly with someone who is very special to you.

Men are particularly prone to extra-high anxiety the first time they go to bed with a new partner. If you keep in mind the very common male fear about "getting it up and keeping it up," you'll begin to see that his anxieties are probably even more intense than yours. However, *both* of you can be more relaxed about "the first time" if you concentrate on the following:

Reassure him that you'll have complete privacy.

One of the big fears that men have is that a husband or boyfriend or child will barge in and discover what's going on in the bedroom. Tell him that no one is coming home, or, if anyone is expected, tell him truthfully what time he or she will be arriving. If you have small children in the house, inform him of their presence and make sure that he sees you locking the door to the bedroom. When you reassure him about the state of privacy in the house, also point out the bathroom in case he'd like to use it.

Start by suggesting a bath or massage.

(More about relaxing massages in the next chapter.)

Keep your sense of humor.

It's pretty certain that both of you are going to touch the wrong spots, do the wrong things, make clumsy movements, so accept your nervousness with a sense of humor. One man told me that he was making love for the first time with the woman of his dreams. "We had been in bed for a few minutes when I realized I urgently had to go to the bathroom. We had had Chinese food and ten cups of tea, and at least two or three beers. I worked up the courage to say to her, 'I'm sorry but I have to visit the john right now!' She burst out with, 'Oh, thank God, I do too,' and we began to laugh. From then on, the barriers were down and everything went just fine."

Refuse to be hurried.

Start your lovemaking by setting a leisurely, relaxed pace. For most people the first few times are so quick they don't have a chance to feel anything fully, so refuse to be hurried. He'll appreciate it when he thinks of you later. Even if you are running toward bed dropping your clothes as fast as you can unzip or unsnap them, take the time to light two or three candles to create a seductive atmosphere. Candles are important. Not only do they allow you both to see and read each other's reactions, they give a soft, flattering light that hides figure flaws and makes faces look their best. Candles also tend to slow you down. The light is old-fashioned, romantic, and unhurried. "I have learned to be maddeningly slow when I'm going to bed with a man," says one high-powered fashion editor, "but it's all done on purpose. I usually suggest taking a shower together just as we're about to get down to basics. The tension builds and it's much more of a turn-on."

No fast or sudden moves.

Keep all your movements fluid and sensual. An unexpected or quick motion can take him by surprise and cause him an anxious moment, disturbing the sensual, relaxed atmosphere. "If a woman caresses me slowly, I tend to think she's not uptight and that she's enjoying herself. I think of quick touches as nervous ones," points out one man.

Also try and keep your caresses fluid. For example, don't explore his chest and suddenly touch his penis. Work your way down, keeping constant tactile touch either by kissing or by soft stroking. Don't suddenly reach up to turn on a light so that you can find some lotion or lubricant. Gently tell him you're going to turn on a light if you haven't already lit candles.

Understand "performance anxiety."

The following version of a very common bedtime story was told to me by a thirty-six-year-old woman from Cleveland named Marcia. "Everything was perfect: the time, the place, the man. Elliot was someone I had known for months, had worked with occasionally (he supplies free-lance art work to the agency I work for), and was attracted to. We'd been out casually as a couple but had never been more intimate than a good-night kiss. This was our first 'real' date and it was storybook: a movie that we both laughed over, a dinner in a small romantic restaurant with soft music and candles. We could hardly wait to get back to my place for the inevitable. Before I could put the chain lock on the door we were in each other's arms. Kissing Elliot was incredibly exciting, and I could feel he was excited too. Within minutes we were undressed and in bed. That's when the trouble began. As much as I knew he wanted to, he couldn't. I could feel that he was horribly embarrassed. This had never happened to me before. The relationship ended right there because I wasn't equipped to deal with the situation."

Marcia and Elliot's problem is a very common one, and like Marcia, few women know how to handle it. Assuming that Elliot's problem was a form of the first-time jitters and not a more deep-rooted problem, there *are* several things a woman can do.

First, your partner may be a man who has difficulty having an erection unless he is stroked directly on the penis. Try some soft, gentle, unfrenzied stroking of his penis with your hand or your mouth. If after a few minutes he doesn't respond or if you sense he seems even more anxious, then stop what you're doing (make it as unabrupt as possible) and just go on kissing and caressing other parts of his body. Don't become anxious yourself and jump out of bed. Just remain as relaxed as possible, keeping the following in mind. You should be aware that the man who has difficulty in attaining an erection and is unresponsive to a few minutes of direct stimulation is faced with anxiety about making love. The question that *you* must face is how to alleviate that anxiety.

Usually, the most effective way to deal with temporary impotence due to performance anxiety is to use a nondemanding, nonthreatening approach and take the attention off performing (meaning, take his mind off an erection). Focus on something else, such as massage or mutual, relaxed stroking of the body: a relaxed, nonanxious, unhurried attitude works wonders. Another way to deal with the situation is to put a man at his ease by recognizing his problem and saying, "It's not important. Why don't we just relax, there's always tomorrow." If you say words to this effect — and you *mean* them — it does a great deal to alleviate his anxiety. He won't feel miserably rejected, because you've assured him that you want to see him again. Often if you both forget about lovemaking for a while and are just warm and affectionate, you'll find he has a spontaneous erection. Don't make a big issue of it, however. Any focus on an erection can make an anxious man lose it. The best thing to do is take it slow and let him set the pace. Do *not* ever hurry him into penetration.

There are differing degrees of performance anxiety, ranging from the first-night jitters to a deep-rooted impotence. Chapter 13 discusses ways to deal with the more serious kinds of erection problems that can paralyze a relationship.

For a woman, performance anxiety is a relatively new phenomenon that has come about with all the emphasis about achieving the "Big O" or "Multiple O's." Performance anxiety for women usually means a fear of being unable to reach orgasm. When you're making love with a man for the first time, or even the first few times, you probably won't have an orgasm. Reaching a satisfying climax usually takes time and effort and involves both verbal and nonverbal communication. However, the second or third time that you're in bed with him, *talk* with him about what feels good for each of you. One friend of mine says, "It's easier to tell someone you don't know very well what you want or how you feel. I've found myself at a party telling a relative stranger intimate things about my life that I would find very hard to tell my husband." Take advantage of the newness of the relationship and begin, at the early stages, to tell him what you want and ask what he wants. More on how to do this in an upcoming chapter.

No faking, please.

Don't fake pleasure and don't fake an orgasm. It's going to backfire on you in the long run. Pretending to like what your partner is doing to or with you means slamming the door on your own enjoyment. He'll never learn what really turns you on if you fake, and though he may not see directly through your deception he'll eventually sense that something is wrong and question the relationship. "My husband thought he was a great lover," says one woman, "until he had an affair with a woman who let him know he was not, and taught him what he needed to know. I had always supported the idea that he was one of the world's greatest lovers and that I was ecstatically happy with his efforts. He was deeply hurt by my pretense — and justifiably angry — we narrowly escaped a breakup. I ended up learning a very basic lesson and also learning what sex was about, for the first time."

NINE

The Geisha's Secret

At precisely five minutes to five a blonde woman in a dark, luxurious fur coat and knee-high leather boots enters a red-lacquered door on Fifth Avenue in Manhattan. The elevator attendant with his immaculate white gloves presses a button and within seconds she is whisked eight floors up into a room with a deep rich carpeting and pale pink walls. The furniture is restrained and elegant. There is a hush about the room.

The blonde woman gives her name to one of the two perfectly coiffed women at a lacquered desk and is handed a small key on a silken cord.

She heads to the left, down a hall with many doors, each one mirrored. Unlocking one, she enters a small room and undresses, slipping out of her pale peach sweater and skirt without haste. Nude, she places her pedicured feet into a pair of slippers and wraps a pink robe around her.

She enters another smallish room. In the center

is a table covered with deep padding and swathed with white sheets and a featherweight blanket.

Another woman, in a pink uniform, is waiting in the room. Without speaking, the blonde takes off her robe and lies back on the table. A hot-water bottle wrapped in a pink towel is placed under her feet. "Now," says the woman in the uniform, her voice discreet and subdued, "you will please lie on your stomach," and she takes some pale lotion and warms it between her hands: the massage is about to begin.

•

Every day, Monday through Friday, at a well-known beauty salon in New York, the famously rich, the not-so-rich, and the highly sensual enter through a lacquered red door on Fifth Avenue and spend an hour with a trained masseuse.

Why have a massage? What is the mystique that makes people say that a massage is one of the most pleasurable and relaxing experiences one can have after a difficult or physically strenuous day? "A good massage," says the chief psychiatrist at one New York hospital, "can help to evaporate the tensions of the body and mind — it can make you feel newborn."

These are not the only benefits — a massage is also one of the great secrets of great lovemaking. The benefits of massage as a prelude to making love have been known for centuries, but it was Masters and Johnson who actually underscored their importance for couples today. In Masters and Johnson's clinics, couples who are brought through the various stages of sexual intimacy begin with "nondemanding stroking" of the back, face, the arms, the legs. This kind of relaxing, nondemanding, nonthreatening stroking is simply a variation or combination of massage techniques that anyone can do.

You should be familiar with two kinds of massage. The first, the relaxing or Swedish massage, as it is often called, is usually administered by a licensed professional. In order to grasp fully what is involved, ask your physician or orthopedist to recommend a good masseur or masseuse and arrange to have a Swedish massage. If you live in a large city you may find beauty salons or health clubs that have on-staff professionals. If you ask at the beginning of a session, most masseurs will gladly take a few minutes at the end to show you the basic strokes they've been using. (Prices usually range from about fifteen to forty dollars an hour.)

The second type of massage can be given by anyone and definitely needs no special professional training. Known as the "sensuous massage," it simply involves long, smooth, loving, caring strokes, light pounding, kneading, and rubbing of all parts of the body. The sensuous massage can often end in pre-sex.

I've found in talking to men that what they prefer is a combination of the muscle-relaxing and the sensuous massage. One man explained why by pointing out that stroking and rubbing are "basically affectionate gestures. When you add manipulation of the muscles, you're adding relaxation, plus you feel right away that a woman knows how to handle your body."

There are many reasons why this kind of massage is such an important and effective tool for making love. When you suggest "a back rub," you alleviate the awkward problems of how to begin touching each other's bodies. "An older woman put me on to massage," says John, a good-looking young carpenter. "I was very attracted to this woman, but I wasn't sure what moves to make with her. . . . I had finished some bookshelves at her house and we were sitting around drinking iced tea. She asked if my muscles were sore and would I like a back rub. Things just naturally developed from there."

Besides helping to combat embarrassment, massage is an excellent means of learning to use and accept your own body and his. It's also the easiest way to begin to explore your partner's body to find out where and how he likes to be touched.

Many people are nervous about accepting pleasure and are often not aware of their anxiety. They feel it's perfectly okay to give pleasure and to touch, but they're inhibited or feel guilty about accepting what feels good. Men (and women) who are shy and find it difficult to "let go" often respond very well to the idea of massage, since it helps quell their anxieties or fears about pleasure. In a massage situation they are *supposed* to accept sensual pleasure, and thus they often feel less guilty about it.

Massage also takes the emphasis away from performance. The man who has trouble attaining an erection will be grateful to the woman who takes the focus off his penis and starts out by rubbing his back or kneading the tension knots out of his hands and feet. Since massage is not an explicit sexual activity, it does not have to lead to making love. Massage can be a pleasurable end in itself, and a massage session can be an unthreatening introduction to direct lovemaking at another time.

How do you begin a massage? You might just stand behind his chair if he's reading or watching television and start to work out the tension spots in the back of his neck, but for a serious massage you'll need to move to a bed. Ask him where he feels the most tension. Most people feel tightness in the shoulders, the neck, and the upper and lower back, so even if he doesn't give you any specific leads, start with one of these areas. Turn off any direct lights and slip your hands under his shirt so that you are in direct contact with his skin. After a while, if you feel it's appropriate, ask him to take his shirt off so that you can work on the rest of his back.

Ideally you'll use lotion or oil, a slippery kind with "play" in it, meaning it doesn't dry out too quickly. Nutraderm, Lubriderm, and Vaseline Intensive Care are all good, and they're nonoily. If you're going to use a lotion with a fragrance in it, check with him first to see if he likes it.

Professionals prefer using oils and often work with ones that have apricot, peppermint, or other light natural fragrances as a base. Baby oil is another choice of some professionals. Still others work with mineral oil. One well-known masseur that I interviewed says, "I use at most two or three tablespoons of oil for the entire body. Most novices use too much and lose control of their movements."

Many men don't like the feel of oil against their skin. They're not as familiar with body lotions as women are, so rub some of whatever you're using on the back or palm of his hand to get him used to the feeling of it. Do not pour oil or lotion directly onto his skin: it's too cool and impersonal. Warm the lotion in your hands first.

There are many different strokes or movements that a professional masseur or masseuse uses. The most common are kneading, pressing with the heels of both hands, pressing with the thumbs alone, lightly beating with the edges of your hands (from the edge of the wrist downward along the little finger), and rapid rubbing strokes that warm the skin with friction. "My best advice to beginners," says Frank Bosco, another highly respected masseur, "is to start with long slow stroking over the entire back." This extended stroking gives you a good feel for the body and you can go on from there, imitating as best you can the motions you've learned under the trained hands of a professional. You'll be able to invent your own style of stroking and kneading as you become more proficient.

Take your time and make steady, consistent, fluid movements. The object of a massage at this stage is to relax the body, not to make its owner sexually aroused. Music can be a great help. Slow, easy sounds are very relaxing and help you to stroke in an

80

even, steady, flowing rhythm. As much as possible keep your hands on his body at all times. Try to remain in constant physical touch with him even when you shift position or pour oil (pour it into your cupped hand resting on his body).

The first stage of a massage skirts any of the erogenous zones. Work on the back first, then move with caressing strokes from the back of the head down the back to the buttocks, down the legs to the feet and toes. As you're doing this, ask where it feels best, ask what kind of pressure he likes, firm, light, heavy.

Then suggest that he turn over and begin to repeat on the front of his body, whatever movements he seemed to enjoy, working upward from the feet toward the head, avoiding the genitals.

Some of the newer sex manuals from the West Coast stress the importance of the flow of breath for total sexual release and enjoyment. As you massage, you might try practicing this special kind of "let go" breathing: take long, deep breaths by first exhaling slowly and then inhaling slowly through your nose, letting your abdomen expand to the utmost. These deep "letting go" breaths, it is said, serve to "energize" your entire sexual system.

Once you've relaxed the tension and worked the muscles, then you can begin to combine your movements with more specifically erotic ones if you feel you're both ready. At this point boundaries between massage and pre-sex are blurred. When you come to specifically erogenous zones, including the penis, stroke or rub them in exactly the same manner that you do the rest of the body, but with less pressure and a very light touch.

Some experts and therapists recommend keeping track of your fantasies while you are giving this kind of massage and suggesting to your husband or lover that he do the same. You can discuss your fantasies afterward and this encourages more openness, more imaginative lovemaking, and even further breaking down of barriers caused by anxiety or tension.

After you have finished his massage you can ask for a reciprocal one if he hasn't already offered, or you might suggest taking a warm shower or bath, but more likely you'll find yourselves very much wanting to go on and make love. . . .

TEN

Bedtime Detective Work

D ON'T TOUCH! That's what we learned when we were kids, and some of us are still following those orders. Men in our society rarely touch each other except in athletic games, most married couples touch each other less and less as time goes by, and it's a long-standing joke about how chic women often just kiss the air instead of touching the cheek that's dutifully offered to them at dinner parties. Research has shown that babies must be touched often and with caring, loving hands in order to thrive, sometimes even to survive. We all need to be touched to reaffirm that we're human, we're alive, we're loved.

Says a friend of mine who claims he can discover if a woman is good in bed simply by her touch, "A woman who is competent sexually usually has a firm but gentle touch. She's deft, doesn't flutter. She places her hand on your arm and holds it there for a second or two longer than the nonsensual/sexual woman does."

Our most sensitive areas are the erogenous zones (literally, "love-producing areas," from the Greek words *eros*, meaning "love," and *gignesthai*, to "be born"). Responses in the erogenous zones differ with different people because of their physical and psychological backgrounds, but warm, full lovemaking can help to develop erotic or love-producing sensitivity in almost any part of the body.

Kissing is one of the best ways to track down erogenous areas. Just by kissing a man on the mouth you can discover some important clues about him. How do his lips respond to your kiss? Are his lips taut or relaxed and open? Does he use his tongue in places you don't expect: for instance, tracing the front of the gums between the teeth and the upper lip, the highly sensitive roof of the mouth? Does he then go on to kiss you in the ear? Does he gently bite the muscles of your neck? Does he kiss your hands? If he does some, any, or all of these, the chances are that the areas he's concentrating on are the places on his own body that respond highly to touching and kissing, that is, they're erogenous zones for him. There's an important principle at work here: in bed you often give what you really want to get for yourself. So observe what he does to you very carefully. He's providing basic clues about what gives him pleasure.

If he's relatively unsophisticated about kissing — you'd be surprised how many people are — you should take the initiative and kiss him on the mouth, on the neck, the ears. Try kissing him on other parts of his body, places that he might not expect. Kissing the hands, for instance, can be highly erotic. Try licking and kissing between the fingers or holding one of his fingers in your mouth.

A good kiss is concentrated, moist, warm, well placed. A bad kiss is bruising, mushy, sloppy.

Another interesting way to track down erogenous zones is to find out where he's ticklish. If you can locate the areas where he's ticklish — backs and tops of knees, armpits, bottoms of feet, anywhere that he reacts strongly — you know that these are zones that are vulnerable and will probably be responsive to very gentle, nonticklish kissing, licking, and stroking. "I go crazy when someone tickles me," one man told me. "My girl friend knows this, and one night she tickled and kissed me at the same time. I can only describe the feeling as somewhere between pleasure and pain, with the pleasure winning out. A little later, I had the most intense climax I'd ever had."

Often men themselves aren't aware that a whole world of feeling exists in places other than the penis; that there are love-producing zones all over the body. Some men know what specific areas are turn-on places for them but are too shy or too timid about letting their partner know what feels especially good. You'll find that most men are highly responsive in the following erogenous areas:

The ears.

One of the most undiscovered spots of pleasure for men (as well as women) is the ear. Lightly circling the inner rims of his ear with your tongue is highly erotic. For the most intense feeling, make your tongue very pointed and slip the tiny end of it into the deepest part of the ear, making quick in-and-out motions that simulate the in-and-out movement of intercourse. Blowing (lightly) into the ear after you have done this feels good, too.

The neck.

The muscles and tendons at the side of the neck are especially sensitive. Many men respond quite intensely to soft biting or massaging of these tendons, which stretch from behind each ear down to the top of the shoulders.

The armpits.

For many men this is a secret area of great erotic sensitivity. Stroke or kiss or softly bite under the arms and along the muscle that leads down the side of his body from the outer edge of the armpit.

The nipples.

Fifty to sixty percent of males have either a partial or a full erection of the nipples when they are stimulated. The stimulation of a man's nipples is slightly different from that of a woman's in that the feeling for him is more direct, more specific, and usually more fleeting. For a man, the best kind of sensation comes from kissing, sucking, or rolling the nipples. The entire surface of the chest does not seem to be as sensitive as a female's.

The buttocks.

Soft biting or gentle pinching of the buttocks can be exciting to most males. The most pleasurable sensations can come from kissing or biting the buttocks while directly stimulating the penis at the same time. Some men also respond to a feathery touching of the tiny hairs above the tailbone and a soft pressure from the base of the spine and up the spinal column for three or four inches.

The inner surfaces of the thighs.

From the penis and scrotum on down to about the middle of the upper leg — the area where his inner thighs would touch a saddle — is highly sensitive. Men particularly respond to light biting or firm kissing of the muscles or tendons in the upper areas, near the genitals, and to licking, kissing, or light massaging of the entire area.

The penis.

There is one basic area of the body that you can count on as certain to bring strong sensation to a man, and that is his penis. Most women know this, but many don't know the exact spots on the penis that give the most intense sensation.

The last inch of the penis, including the head, is the area of greatest sensitivity. Stimulating the very delicate vertical thread of skin on the underside of the penis that joins the head to the shaft gives the absolute maximum of sensation (apparently equivalent to the feeling a woman has when her clitoris is stimulated). The long ridge, which can look like an engorged vein, that runs along the underside of the penis is also an area of high sensation.

Most men like the penis to be stroked or held firmly. But "firm" to you might be "timid" to him. Don't make the mistake of equating how you would like your clitoris or vaginal area to be touched with the way he would like to be touched genitally. One man likened the difference in touch between penis and vagina by saying, "It's like comparing a pneumatic drill and a soufflé. It takes a certain amount of strength and experience to handle the drill properly, but with a soufflé you need a delicacy of touch that takes skill as well as experience."

Finding out how firmly he wants to be touched comes only through trial and error, but you should keep in mind that the head of the penis is the most sensitive area and responds to varying degrees of touch. The shaft has much less feeling to it; you can grip or clasp it with more strength. Men say most women do not hold the penis firmly enough when they are moving the outside skin of the penis up and down. "A good feel" was described by one man as one that is somewhere between "holding a tennis racquet and grasping a pot handle." Often, when stroking or clasping a penis, you'll find that your partner will respond even more to a slight tightening of the fingers as they descend toward the base of the penis.

Scrotum and anus.

The skin of the scrotum is highly sensitive and responds to licking and kissing. Also try blowing out short, light breaths directly to the skin surface. Another especially erotic area lies between the base of the scrotum and extends to the anus. Many men feel that, after the penis, the anus is the next most erogenous area on the body.

There are two crucial don'ts about touching a man's genital area. Don't apply more pressure to the penis and/or scrotum when he is in the throes of climax. It may distract and/or cause him discomfort. And don't ever grasp his testicles tightly because that is *sure* to make him wince with pain.

•

The above listing includes all the well-documented erogenous zones but almost any part of the body can qualify. Stay keenly alert so you'll know when you've hit one of your lover's sensitive, responsive areas. His whole body or part of it may react by a slight stiffening, he may breathe a little more deeply or audibly sigh, or his hands and toes may stiffen and curl very slightly. Sometimes the palms and the soles of his feet will become moist if he is being erotically stimulated in a particularly sensitive place. Some men also display a pale pink to red flush over the chest when they are extremely stimulated.

One last thought to keep well in mind: don't ever confuse a firm touch with a grabby touch. Men, as well as women, react very negatively to this kind of pawing. Quick, grabby movements are not conducive to making love. Generally speaking, slow, even, caressing movements are far better. You should begin with these and then slowly and gradually work up to firmer and firmer stroking, again keeping in mind that not only your hands but every part of your body can touch and be touched in return.

ELEVEN

Making Love to a Man

I t seems to me that women spend far more time learning how to cook than they do learning how to make love. Mastering the art of the soufflé seems to take precedence over developing skill and knowledge of the simple technical aspects of the sex act. When you make love to a man you want to give him a complete experience, one that is totally pleasurable. In the physical sense, this means that you are trying to give him not just an ejaculation but a full, intense orgasm. One man described the difference this way: "One kind of coming is centered in my groin, which is a hot, specific, releasing feeling, but the other kind of coming, which I think is like a woman's orgasm, feels like fireworks. The rockets go off in my penis and a shower of spasms spreads all through my body." The keys to giving a man this kind of physical sensation lie in *timing* and specific *techniques* that can be easily learned by any woman.

Timing: The Crucial Factor

Somehow many women have the notion that they should attain an orgasm according to a stopwatch and that a man should reach his climax fairly quickly — and that's that. This may derive from the fact that, historically, "nice" or "good" women were expected to be passive and let the male come to a speedy climax. Some women also feel that they must have an orgasm before their partner ejaculates, another "must" that is unjustified. These attitudes contribute to hurried, uncaring sex. Another reason that many of us tend to make love in minimal time is that we are on rushed, often frenzied schedules. Today, not only do many of us care for the children, cook, clean, keep ourselves in shape, argue with the mechanic about new mufflers, we also contribute to the family income. Husbands or lovers are under equal pressure. It's not surprising that by ten-thirty at night most people are in a state close to exhaustion, and although you may want to make love, you may both have a tendency to speed things up so you can get enough sleep to take you through the next crowded day.

"Most Americans make love as if they're running a race," points out one sex expert. "You can certainly have an exciting, quick sexual encounter, but most women are unaware that to really make love to a man requires time." It takes very little time for a man simply to ejaculate, but it takes an extended amount of time to give a man the intense kind of orgasm that differentiates lovemaking from plain routine sex.

Physiologically, the more stimulation that a man experiences, the more intense and dramatic his orgasm or climax will be. The sexually knowledgeable woman will physically prolong a man's erection and delay his ejaculation so that he (as well as she) can experience an orgasm in its ultimate intensity. *Neither* of you can be hurried if you want to know what a thundering orgasm is like — for both of you.

Most women prefer nonstop genital stimulation that builds up to an orgasm, but men can be stimulated to a point just short of climax, the stimulation stopped for at least several seconds, then resumed. The buildup and slowdown process is what gives the extraordinary intensity to an orgasm. For most men, a building up/slowing down can be achieved two or more times. Three or four or even more cycles are possible. Some men, however, report that they have difficulty in having an orgasm if they are brought to the brink too many times. Try it once or twice at first, and then go on longer when you both know each other's rhythms more specifically. Ask him if he is near the point of ejaculation so that you'll know when to stop. If you are in a position to see or feel his genitals, you can often tell when a climax is near because the scrotum has become compact and wrinkled and has begun to ascend toward the body cavity.

There is a special technique used by knowledgeable lovers to help to prevent or slow ejaculation. Called the squeeze technique, it can help to build up an exquisite tension. However, it requires your utmost sensitivity and *must be employed with caution and only with the cooperation of your partner*. If your partner is interested in trying the squeeze technique, ask him to tell you when he's reaching the point of no return. As he is coming to a climax, his testicles, which usually hang at rest in the scrotum, begin to ascend toward the body cavity and the scrotum becomes contracted and wrinkled, forming a firm rounded mass. Take your thumb and forefinger and encircle the top of his scrotum, making sure that the testicles are below the ring of your fingers. Gently squeeze or tighten your thumb and index finger together and at the same time apply a pressure toward his body with your entire hand. The pressure should be quite firm. Ask your husband or lover what pressure works for him. The right amount of pressure for about six to ten seconds should effectively stop an ejaculation. However, if an orgasm has begun, don't try to stop it. "If a woman waits until a man is coming and then stops what she is doing, he will have the orgasm without direct stimulation and this can be one of the most unsatisfying experiences a man can have sexually," points out an experienced single man.

Remember that you can stop an ejaculation either by the squeeze technique or simply by stopping all your movements, one or more times, in order to heighten a climax. Once you have retarded a climax you can go back and continue what you've been doing, switch to something else like the missionary position, or oral sex, or take an even longer break to have a glass of wine or put a record on. For most men, a delay, if it's timed just right, can be the prelude to an extraordinary orgasm.

You might find that some men may resist prolonged lovemaking at first because they are not familiar with the build up/slow down process, and they may simply want to follow their old habits of coming quickly to a climax. Once, however, you both experience this extended kind of lovemaking, which gives such an intensified range of sensations and feeling, you will probably want to experience it again and again.

Beyond delay, there are two specific techniques you can learn that help a man feel as if he's had a "fireworks" orgasm: (1) the woman-on-top position; (2) oral sex.

Woman-on-top Position

This particular position is one of the great secrets of making love to a man. It prolongs the physical act, gives intense stimulation to the woman, and helps her control her partner's climax so that it becomes most heightened.

Some women say that they are reluctant to suggest this position because they feel they might appear overly aggressive. On the contrary, for many men this is the most erotic way to make love. One man observes, "When a woman is on top of me I can see and feel everything. There is something fantastic about holding and watching a woman who is turned on." Another man echoed many opinions when he said, "Never underestimate the power of visual effects for a man. If she's astride, she is there for me to *see*, and she's there for me to *love*."

The *Kama-Sutra*, a text on the art of sex and love written seventeen centuries ago, advises that a woman should give a man

. . . assistance by acting his part. . . . There are two ways of doing this, the first is when during congress she turns round and gets on top of her lover, in such a manner as to continue the congress, without obstructing the pleasure of it; and the other is when she acts the man's part from the beginning. At such a time, with flowers in her hair hanging loose, and her smiles broken by hard breathings, she should press upon her lover's bosom with her own breasts, and lowering her head frequently, should do in return the same actions which he used to do before.

Woman Astride Step-by-Step

As he lies on his back, kneel over his body. Your knees and feet are on the bed, on the outside of his thighs, and you are kneeling astride him, facing him. Support your weight evenly on both legs. You will probably need one or both of your hands for leverage; they should be on his chest, or you can clasp or intertwine hands over his chest for further support. Very gently and slowly insert his erect penis into you. You should have no lubrication problems if you've used lotion or oil during massage. If you need some lubricant, apply it directly to his penis.

Now the pelvic movements that were described in Chapter 6 begin. If you have practiced, you will be able to use several different motions. You can rotate your pelvis and grip with your interior muscles as you move up and down on his penis. Or you can grip while you are sliding back and forth toward his shoulders. Some women can control the penis to such a degree that they can "flip" the head against the cervix to amplify the pleasurable sensations to an extreme. Some manuals point out that you can rotate 180 degrees and face his feet, but many men feel that they can't see or touch as much and, as one man put it, this is "wasted effort."

When you are sitting astride a man's pelvis and his penis is erect inside you, the feeling for him is like a lapping or stroking or licking rather than the clasped, concentrated sensations that he feels when he's on top. The opening to the vagina is wider than when you are supine with your legs closer together. This widening makes the physical feelings less intense for him, but the sensations are usually still sufficient for him to maintain his erection. He is not in much danger of coming to an early climax because of the difference in the movements of stroking and thrusting, and he is able to be more relaxed because he is on his back. He can, of course, partake as much as he wants by thrusting his pelvis to meet your movements, or by moving you back and forth as he places his hands on your hips and guides you. Or, like many men, once he gets used to the idea, he can lie back, watch, and enjoy what you're doing.

The woman-astride position usually gives the greatest degree of penetration to you and also allows your most sensitized areas to be in direct contact with the man's genitals for the most heightened sensations. Specifically, this means that your clitoris and the erogenous areas surrounding and including the vagina are receiving a high degree of stimulation. Your husband or lover may want to intensify these feelings even more by manually stimulating your clitoris and your breasts. Your amplified reactions make him, in turn, even more responsive.

When you're on top, you can roll over while he's still inside you, if you take your time and adjust your bodies slowly and carefully, to the "missionary" position. Try this for a while and then switch back to being on top or to oral sex, always being sensitive to an impending climax on his part. If he indicates he's about to have an orgasm and you both wish to further prolong lovemaking, you can stop for a few moments completely, and then work up to a crescendo again. Don't try too much at one time — too many positions in one session can make either or both of you feel you're trying out for a sort of sexual Olympics.

Some women find they can fairly easily come to orgasm when they are astride a man because the stimulation to the clitoris is so intense. If you do have an orgasm, another advantage to the on-top position is that the man may be able to feel the contractions of your vagina, which of course stimulates him even further. "One of the reasons I love my wife to be on top," said one man, "is that I can feel her contracting around me because I'm not pressing down or thrusting, and I'm just in a relaxed position open to feeling everything that's going on. She can have as many orgasms as she wants and I still don't come — until we both sense it's the right time."

Oral Sex

In a *Redbook* 1980 survey of more than 26,000 men and women, the amount of times that a couple has sex is "the topic most argued about." The next most argued-about topic is oral sex. One of the key observations of the survey was that "among women, a higher proportion who said they liked oral sex rated their sexual relationship as good or excellent." Remember, however, that you don't have to like oral sex in order to have a good sex life, the authors conclude; rather, "you have to be able to tell your partner what you like and what makes you uncomfortable."

The Joy of Sex notes that oral sex, once taboo, is now almost obligatory. But no matter how obligatory it is, many women are still highly uncomfortable with it. Perhaps the most effective way to deal with the problem is to tell your husband or lover how you feel. A frank discussion can do wonders to clear up misinformation, misconceptions, and possible stored-up resentments. Oral sex is certainly not an obligation, but before you count it out altogether you might want to know why men feel it is so important.

Almost without exception the men I talked with voiced a lack of satisfaction in the area of oral sex. Many men complain that although women are becoming more eager to accept oral sex because they think it's the thing men want, they don't really understand its importance, they don't really know how to do it well, and they are timid about learning. "I enjoy oral sex from my husband," declared one woman who has been married two years, "but I'm not really quite sure what I'm doing when it comes to him. I'm too embarrassed to ask my husband how to do it now."

Recent informal surveys indicate that oral sex is the most-asked-for service from professionals. Oral sex *is* important to most men, whether they admit it openly or not. Men, as well as society in general, feel that the penis is symbolic of their masculinity. The majority of men want women to acknowledge their maleness by accepting the penis on a physical and emotional level, and by becoming involved with it in an open, joyful, nonanxious way. Not only does this symbolize an acceptance and acknowledgment of a man's sexuality, but oral sexual experiences can be, to some males, as intimate and meaningful as penetrating a woman's vagina.

Even though oral sex has significant emotional connotations for many men, there are also very specific physical reasons why it is so important to making love. You have far more control of your mouth and your hands than you do of your vagina. Your mouth and hands can give your partner a variety of exquisite sensations that can repeatedly bring him to the brink of climax. By using oral techniques, you don't just rely on the in-and-out thrusting of penis/vagina to give him pleasure. You have the control and can play upon a complete spectrum of your husband's or lover's responses to give him maximum sensation. One man put it this way: "Oral sex is the intensification of all the feelings one has being inside a woman. But everything feels even more specific. When combined or alternated with genital sex, oral stimulation can be one of the most valuable physical ways of bringing someone to the most terrific climax he can have."

By using oral techniques, you can first stimulate and arouse him and then duplicate all the feelings he has when he's inside you, and give him even more of a variety of sensations. Your mouth can make a tight, vaginalike passage for his penis; it can also suck in or out. Your lips can kiss in a myriad of ways. Your tongue can give an almost infinite variety of sensations depending on whether you keep it pointed, or flat, or round. Your lips can nip, lick, trace. Your hands can make endless movements to caress and stimulate his genitals and they can work with your mouth to give the maximum of feeling. These are some of the pleasures of sophisticated oral sexuality.

"Oral sex," observes a highly experienced woman, "does not just have to do with mouth and cock. It has to do with placing something in your mouth. A penis works best, but toes, eyelashes, fingers also make for incredibly exciting feelings. I used to read about these things in sex manuals and I thought it was just so many words, but I tried them and they work. I really do think of my mouth as an instrument that can be used to delight, distract, delay, and intensify my husband's climaxes."

If you're uncomfortable about oral sex but are willing to try, take it one small step at a time. Most men will be appreciative and tell you it's worth the effort, and that alone should help to motivate you.

Oral Sex Step-by-Step

If you've read any literature on oral sex, you'll probably come away with the feeling that it involves a fairly simple physical movement. It does and it doesn't. You can suck on a penis, naturally, easily, and quickly. However, good or skillful oral sex is more complicated. There's no magic involved; sucking is a natural response, but refinements can be learned. It's these refinements that make the big difference between the kindergarten variety of sex and the sophistication of graduate-school lovemaking.

There are two mental secrets to expert oral sex. These are simply that you must want, above all, to give your man pleasure, and you must learn to concentrate completely on what you're doing.

Learning oral sex is a little like learning how to swim. First you have to take the *risk* of getting into water and learning to keep afloat. Applying this to oral sex means that you have to make up your mind that you *want* to do it, and then begin. Next, in swimming, you've got to remember your breathing, your kicking, your stroke, your speed. In oral sex you need to remember to move up and down with your mouth, remember your timing, control your touch, and coordinate your hand movements to your mouth movements. Once you've mastered the basics — and they are fairly easy — you may want to advance further and really perfect your technique. Nature is on your side: these are instinctive, natural movements and will come to you with just a little practice. One of the best things you can do is to *ask* your husband or lover to guide your head and/or your mouth with his own hand so that you get the rhythm and stroking feeling correct for his particular preferences. After a few times, basic technique becomes automatic and you can begin to work on perfecting that technique into real expertise.

This is important to remember: *all motions should be done continuously*. You wouldn't want him to stop stroking you on the clitoris when you're intensely stimulated, so be just as considerate of him.

Now, think of your mouth as the opening of a vagina and think of your hands as an extension of your mouth. Begin by licking his penis with your tongue. Make your tongue as sharp and pointed as you can and use it to probe gently the areas around the most sensitive part, the head. If, at this point, you begin to have thoughts that this is dirty or unpleasant or you are anxious, control your mind and try and *concentrate totally* on what you are doing.

Focus your mind on pointing your tongue, and begin to lick and stroke the penis, concentrating on the ridge that runs down the center of the underside. Go fairly slowly and you'll probably be able to feel the ridge with your tongue. Lightly flick your tongue back and forth on the little ridge of skin where the head is joined to the shaft — for most men this is absolutely the most sensitive and responsive part of the penis. Relax, remember to breathe, and improvise a bit. You may want to lick or kiss the penis or stroke it lengthwise with your tongue.

Return to where the head and shaft connect. *Take your time*, there's no rush. Make smooth, fluid movements. Now envelope the penis with your mouth. The mouth should be kept wide open, the lips drawn back as far as possible in a tight oval covering the teeth, the penis resting on the tongue. Again, if you are having any mental problems about what you're doing, *concentrate completely* on your physical actions.

The all-important oral friction now begins in which your mouth and tongue imitate the reciprocal motion and kneading action of the vagina. Move your mouth back and forth, up and down on the penis, constantly keeping in mind that your lips should feel like a very snug vagina. Begin slowly and increase your speed subtly at every forward stroke.

There is some controversy about what is more important in oral sex. Some men contend that the more length taken into the mouth, the more satisfying it is to them. Others feel that the head of the penis is the most sensitive area and the mouth need cover only that area plus one or two inches down the shaft. If your husband or lover is in this latter contingent, then use one of your hands as an extension of your mouth. Take your thumb and forefinger and make a snug circle around the penis, keeping your mouth touching or nearly touching it. Now move your hand up and down the shaft of the penis in the same rhythm as your mouth. As your mouth goes down onto the shaft, your hand goes downward, too, and vice versa. You can also use your other hand to take care of the exposed parts of the penis, using sensuous, mild finger movements over the shaft and testicles and anal opening.

One of the best and little-known secrets to success here is taking a small amount of body lotion or oil in your hand and applying it to the penis. Many men say saliva is usually not plentiful enough, and the lubricant acts more like your vagina's own secretions, making your hand motions fluid and regular and giving the penis heightened stimulation. Use a *nontasting*, nondrying slippery lotion or oil; Nutraderm was recommended by several men, as was mineral oil. K-Y surgical jelly is also widely used but tends to dry out more quickly. Two women I spoke with said that they didn't like the medicinal taste of lubricants. The problem is usually solved by applying lubricant to the lower shaft of the penis only, the part in contact with your hand.

If your man is one of those who believes in the deep-throat technique, try and get as much of his penis into your mouth as possible. A friend of mine patiently explained that the trick Linda Lovelace used was to throw her head back off the edge of a bed so that her mouth and throat formed one extra-long passage. The amount of penis that can enter your mouth will vary with the size of the penis and with the particular size and shape of your mouth. If you have taken in as much of his penis as you can and you begin the up and down movement, or he begins strong thrusting, you may find that you have a tendency to gag. If you do gag, *don't* fall into a fit of embarrassment — it's a natural response sometimes. Take a second's pause, a deep breath that will relax the muscles, and keep on going. Experience exercises the upper throat and helps eliminate gagging, no matter how hard the thrust.

Once you have begun to move up and down on the penis with your mouth (and hands, if that's what he likes), *take your time* and increase your speed slowly. A true expert at oral sex will intensify the sensations even more by using her hands consistently along with her mouth. This is where your previous detective work comes in. You should, after a few sessions, know what and where feels best to him and use your hands to caress, fondle, nip, stroke, lightly pinch, or trace areas of his body close to his genitals while you are using your mouth. If you're interested in experimenting with different sensations, you might try something as simple as sipping hot tea or cider before you take his penis into your mouth, or try drinking some ice water. Both the hot and cold feelings that are transmitted by your tongue can be interesting new sensations for him.

You can use oral sex as a way of extending lovemaking or as an end in itself. If you are using it as simply one means of stimulation, you would stop before a man comes to a climax and switch to the woman-on-top position or any other position that you are comfortable with. If, however, you both wish to go on to climax you face the question of swallowing the man's ejaculate. Don't do anything that repels you. Some men consider it a very special love sign if a woman is willing to swallow their sperm. Others don't see it as "that big a deal," but it's really a matter of what you feel comfortable with.

Positions

The big difference between genital and oral sex, according to most men, is not physical but emotional. Oral sex can be one of the most loving gifts a woman can give, but genital sex, men say, is ultimately the most fulfilling because there is a feeling of oneness, a bonding, a partaking of each other, a total intimacy.

Genital sex affords an infinite variety of positions for lovemaking that will increase and intensify a man's pleasure. These positions will depend on the way his body — and yours — is constructed. Usually the positions in which he feels the most sensation and the most pleasure are those in which the penis is most snugly fitted into the vagina.

For some men the "missionary" or man-on-top position gives the most pleasurable sensations. Others prefer a front-to-back or rear-entry method. A large group of men say they find the knee-chest position intensely gratifying, and many women agree. Physiologically there are good grounds why this position is a favorite of both sexes. The knee-chest, where the woman's knees are pressed to her chest with her legs extended beyond the man's shoulders, is usually the position where the vagina is most elongated and extended. Thus the penis fits snugly into it. There are other benefits as well. Penetration is much deeper for the man and more pleasurable for the woman, who feels intense friction of the genital area with each thrust.

Every man and woman together must find those positions that give the most amount of penetration, friction, and ultimate pleasure. When you employ these positions, remember to use the prolonging techniques. To put it another way: when you combine the prolonging techniques with the sexual positions that are most pleasurable to you both, you can, as one man poetically put it, "discover the oceanic feeling of bliss and the ecstatic experience of oneness."

TWELVE

Yes, There Are Easy Ways to Talk About Sex

H e makes love in the missionary position most of the time. You'd like to find out what it's like being on top for a while. Can you tell him?

You want him to kiss and touch you there and there and *there*. How do you let him know?

You'd love to make love in a garden under a jacaranda tree by moonlight. Is he aware of your romantic wishes?

You'd like to try anal sex — maybe just once. You could never mention it, could you? (He'd like to try it, too, but forget it — it's too dirty for words, so he doesn't say anything either.)

You'd like to know if *he's* got the same kinds of erotic thoughts on his mind as you do, but how do you ever start up a discussion.

Is there *any* way to talk easily about sex? Every manual, every text, almost every single book on modern sex says that communication is one of the most important parts of lovemaking. "More than any other factor," underscores the *Redbook* sex survey, "effectiveness in conveying one's preferences and feelings about sex is the key to a good sex life." Communicating about sex means that you are revealing your most intimate personal needs, feelings, and wishes, an extremely difficult feat for most of us. But it *is* possible to bring up the subject and to talk about what you both need from each other. Some people will be more direct and straightforward when discussing sex; others will be extremely shy or uncomfortable. The important thing to remember is that no matter what your style or his — direct, subtle, shy, embarrassed — a specific conversation about your needs is essential.

Usually in the first stages of a relationship couples try nonverbal means of telling each other what feels good. Touching and guiding of hands, heads, and bodies is what we typically do to tell each other how we like things to go. Some men and women who know each other well show each other how they like to be stimulated by masturbating in front of their partners — but no matter how enlightening this may prove to be, many couples still feel uncomfortable about doing it. Nonverbal methods work — up to a point — but many of us don't pick up on the clues we're given because they're not clear or specific enough. *Talking,* then, is still the best and most direct way of knowing for sure that his sexual needs, and yours, will be met.

What is the best time and place to talk about sex? Opinions vary widely, but many men I spoke with feel that the easiest place is anywhere but bed. The timing is also very important. Morning seems to be a preferred hour. Explains one articulate lawyer, "I think it's harder to talk about sex when you're in bed. I find Anne and I often slip into a rating system about what happened the last time we made love. We realized that we could have a frank discussion without the scorecard situation more easily in the morning over a cup of coffee in the kitchen." One woman who finds it very difficult to talk about sex says that she can bring up the subject "without too much anxiety" over dinner in an intimate restaurant. "I can talk with more detachment about sex in a public place. It's also a turn-on — for both of us," she says.

Breaking the Ice

How, specifically, can you bring up the subject of sex? The following ideas come from men and women that I interviewed.

"Bring up a controversial issue," advises one woman. "Say something like 'My friend Alison is involved in a three-way, *what* do you think about *that*?' or 'I read somewhere that forty-two percent of men want anal sex but are afraid to ask — do you think that's *true*?' " Once broached, says a friend of mine, "the subject of sex is usually irresistible. . . . It breaks the ice and makes it easy to jump from your opinions and his into specific areas that are of concern to both of you."

Another easy lead-in to a discussion about sex is to ask your husband or lover to read an article or book that you think is provocative or informative. Masters and Johnson's wise and reassuring book, *The Pleasure Bond,* has a wealth of material on the importance of communication, touching, jealousy, fidelity, and many other controversial issues that are at the heart of a relationship. Three clever and useful paperbacks that are tried and true, *The Sensuous Woman, The Sensuous Man, The Sensuous Couple,* all provide interesting take-off points for a discussion of erotic touching, oral sex, anal sex, impotence, bisexuality, and a variety of other topics. They're also easy and amusing to read out loud to your partner just in case he balks at having to do the reading on his own.

Another good approach that works well for someone who is exceptionally shy is one frequently used by actors and actresses when they are appearing in public and have no script to follow. On these occasions, many start off with, "I'm so nervous" — which may or may not be true. Saying this helps, however, to relieve any possible nervousness and gains the audience's sympathy. They often go on to say something like, "It's hard for me to say this . . . ," which also may be true, and is also calculated to get more attention and more sympathy from the audience. Then they usually go on to say what they want to say, in a most effective way.

Asking for Specifics

As I was doing interviews, I found it easier to talk about sexual specifics to men than to women.

They're more open, more comfortable, and they're surprisingly grateful to have the chance to say something about what they want and how they want it. You'll find that most men talk in an unembarrassed way about sex, so if you can get down to details as soon as possible with your husband or lover it will save you a great deal of groping, anxiety, and misunderstanding.

Precisely how do you deal with specifics? Suppose you would like to do something that you haven't tried together before — oral sex or genital kissing, for example — but nothing, so far, has been brought up about the subject? How do you go about saying what you'd like? One highly experienced woman suggests asking a man:

"What do you know that I don't know?"

"This," she says, "is a no-fail method, a sure way of getting him to say what *he* wants. You then can tell him what *you* want. Most men are happy to show off their sexual expertise by teaching you what they think you don't know, and it also gives them the chance to explore things they may have wanted to try but have been afraid to ask."

What if things are getting a bit routine and you'd like to try something new but you don't want to deflate his ego by suggesting that he's not as imaginative or innovative as you'd wish him to be? You might try Helen's solution to the problem. Helen had been married a year when she finally admitted to herself that she was facing a case of the "bedroom blahs.'' Helen is a highly sensual woman who had many lovers before she married Jim. Jim had been brought up in a strictly religious atmosphere and had divorced his first wife (who was his first and only sexual partner) to marry Helen. ''I'm deeply in love with Jim,'' says Helen, ''but I knew I couldn't survive a marriage that was so one-dimensional in the sexual area. Jim was still basically naïve about lovemaking and also very sensitive about the fact that I had been to bed with a lot of men and had done a lot of things. I finally came up with an idea. One Saturday morning when we woke up and were talking in bed I told him I'd had the most exciting dream. I described how he and I were making love on a beach with the water pounding over us, and he was doing the most exciting things to me. Licking me, kissing me, biting me, fucking me in every way I could think of. He was really turned on. It was the beginning of a new phase for us. What he didn't know, and never will, is that I'd lived every one of those experiences.''

You must feel free to express what it is that you want — and also what you don't want. There are often times when you don't feel physically or emotionally like making love when he wants to, and vice versa. Every man and every woman has a different level of sexual drive. In addition, sexual interest changes almost daily. You may be ravenous for sex and he simply isn't. It may have to do with the fact that he has troubles at work or in meeting his financial commitments, or anything at all. Or he may have no visible anxieties at the moment — he's just less interested in sex. Remember when you experienced the same lack of interest. If you have established clear, understanding communication, he should be able to tell you lovingly, without hurting your feelings, that he just isn't in the mood for sex. You should be able to tell him the same thing. It's human, normal, and perfectly okay to be on differing sexual wavelengths. In many instances, if you begin to talk about the way you're feeling, the sexual blocks are resolved and lead to lovemaking. However, if the lack of participation continues for more than ten days or so, on either side, it's wise to discuss it thoroughly with your husband or lover to see if there is any hidden anger or hostility that is causing the problem. If you still can't discover what is causing a lack of sexual interest, it's a good idea to first see a physician and then if necessary, a sexual counselor.

THIRTEEN

Dealing with Erection Problems

Imagine a man with a large light bulb on top of his head that lights up every time he has an erection. When he sees a sexy woman at the office the bulb starts to warm up. When he finds his wife at home in a slinky nightgown, the light gets brighter. When she touches his cock, it's top voltage and that bulb is shining like a beacon. Now imagine the same bedroom scene, light bulb on head, but Nothing Happens. Zip. A complete blackout that you can't miss. That's what it feels like to have an erection problem.

— An executive in a publishing company

There probably isn't a man alive who has not, at some time or another in his life, been unable to have or to keep an erection. Erections, if you remember, are not under a man's control, no matter how fervently he may wish them to be. Anything can stop the action: too much to drink, too much stress, the first-time jitters, an uncaring and unresponsive woman, or a man's just not feeling sexual at the moment. These are occasional or temporary experiences for the majority of men and do not mean that a man is impotent. However, failure to attain an erection can be insidious as well as frightening to a man, particularly if there has been no history of the problem. Suppose he's had a problem for one night and then the same thing happens the next. He begins to worry, the worry escalates to fear that he truly *is* impotent. The fear quickly builds on itself, finally causing a more serious problem, chronic impotence. Obviously it's wise to deal with the situation as soon as possible.

Most men have fairly strong erections on waking and two or three erections during sleep. These men have no physical basis for their erection failures during sex. The small percentage of men with a physical basis for impotence usually do not have these nocturnal or morning erections.

For men with both psychological and physical problems the news is good: Masters and Johnson report curing over half the men they've treated for impotence, and recently important advances have been made in treating and curing the men whose impotence is physiological.

The best way to deal with a man who's had a long-standing problem is to suggest gently that he consider seeing a qualified sex therapist and/or a physician and have a complete physical checkup. To locate a sex therapist, write to: The American Association of Sex Educators, Counselors and Therapists, 5010 Wisconsin Avenue, N.W., Suite 304, Washington, D.C. 20016.

What can you do to help a man with an occasional or recent erection problem? Plenty, if you remember that in his case the failure to have an erection almost always stems from a basic sexual fear: anxiety about performance. In one way or another, the cures that sex experts recommend involve the man's getting into bed with the woman and taking his mind off performing the sexual act.

The first thing you can do is empathize. Most men will be reluctant to discuss the situation, but since there's no way to hide it, it's best to bring the problem out into the open by talking as directly as you can. Reassure him that you can understand how difficult the circumstances are for him. Tell him you're aware of the fears he must be facing and that you can imagine how anxious the situation makes him. Second, work out a plan with him so that he feels no pressure to perform. This is basically the method that Masters and Johnson follow: they bring their patients through "nondemanding stroking" of the back, the face, the arms, the legs (see Chapter 9). The next day they permit manipulation of the breasts and genitals with no intercourse allowed. Fairly soon the man achieves a spontaneous erection, and he is allowed to make use of it in gradual stages. The underlying attitude is relaxed and unthreatening: if a man has an erection, fine; if not, there's always tomorrow.

One man told me that a woman who had been exposed to his impotence for several nights handled the situation by announcing cheerfully and affectionately, "I'm spending the night tonight but we're not going to have sex." "Since I didn't *have* to come up with a hard-on, and was loving and relaxed, it happened automatically," he reported.

Another common way to deal with temporary impotence is limiting yourselves to foreplay every other night. Usually after a week or ten days an erection occurs, but keep in mind that, even though he may have an erection, the focus should still be on caring and sensual stimulation — not performance — until he is having erections fairly regularly.

A friend of mine told me the story of Monique, who had what she charmingly termed "a reluctant lover." "I tried to get him to feel that he was in another world, to defamiliarize him with his surroundings, to make it seem not to be *him* who had to perform," she said. Part of Monique's unique treatment was to talk romantically in French to her reluctant lover, a very clever way of taking his focus off his penis. It worked, and *voilà!* his erection problems disappeared. Monique, a Parisian, claims that there's much truth in the old French saying "There are no impotent men; there are only unskilled women."

FOURTEEN

Sex Shop Escapade

It was one of those steamy, sweltering August days when the most one should be doing is lying back on a chaise longue, lazily eating bonbons and sipping mint juleps, in an air-conditioned drawing room. I, unfortunately, was not in a position to partake of such pleasures. This particular August day found me on the way to the gym resolved to work off the effects of too many cooling Baskin-Robbins binges. While I was walking I also resolved that as soon as I left the gym I'd finish up some essential research that I'd put off doing for far too long.

I made it to the Sheridan Square Health Club and was greeted by Lenny Russell, the club's owner and motivating energy force.

"Hey, the air-conditioning is not doing too well today, but it's better for you that way."

"Thanks, Leonard," I said. "You remind me of my mother; she said that I should always find the good in everything."

A few months before, when I was going to do a story on the best gyms in New York, I had tracked down the knowledgeable Mr. Russell for an interview. Before our talk was over, he told me, "You need to shape up, kid. You can train here."

Thus I became the only woman to exercise at an all-male body builders' gym. By changing into baggy gray sweat pants and sweat shirt in the broom closet, keeping my eyes to the floor, and generally being as small and inconspicuous as possible, I also became privy to an invaluable store of all-male talk. Once Leonard even took me on a sensational whirlwind tour of the crowded locker room. After the "boys" became used to me, I got up the courage to ask some of them if I could have interviews for *How to Make Love to a Man*. The response was invariably an enthusiastic and positive one. So now, in the stifling ninety-degree heat, while trying to do the tortuous exercise program that Leonard had devised for me, I heard, "Hey, Al, how's it going? Finished the book yet?"

"Not yet, not yet. But I should be getting some good information today!" I said nonchalantly. "I'm just on my way up the street to a shop called the Treasure Trove."

"Hey, kid," said Leonard, not registering anything unusual on his face, "whatever turns you on . . ."

"This is serious research, you know," I shot back at him.

"Research, yeah, research. Have a *good* time.

122

And get into the gym *tomorrow*. You think you can shape up at the rate you're going?"

At the rate I'm procrastinating, I thought, I'm never going to get *any*thing done. So I finished my workout and forced myself out into the blazing sun.

I walked the necessary two blocks and arrived at my destination. Peering in, I saw two other shoppers, a man and a woman, in the store, and the young man behind the counter was apparently explaining to the woman how one particular vibrator compared with another. She looked like a normal human being, not a creature from some murky sexual depth. The salespeople, too, appeared reassuringly healthy, as did the other patron, who looked strictly Ivy League and was not wearing the greasy trench coat with turned-up collar that I half expected.

With trepidation I walked into the brightly lighted interior.

"May I help you?" said a clerk, turning to me.

"No thanks, I'm just looking," I replied quite coolly. And indeed there were a great many things to look at that I had never laid eyes on before.

"Perhaps you'd like to glance through the catalog," a young salesperson suggested. This immediately put me at my ease, as I now had something to read that would give me information which I was obviously greatly in need of. While I was skimming the catalog, which was *absolutely fascinating,* I observed the flow of customers. It was about 2:00 P.M., and although not crowded, the shop was doing a brisk business.

In the front of the store, displayed against a tasteful background of gray felt, were postcards, T-shirts, soaps, lotions, and oils. Farther back in the esoteric department were items in rubber and leather, plus straps, rings, masks, bras, pants, belts, and even a pair of chaps.

Finally the store emptied and the clerk turned his full attention to me.

"Is there something special that you were looking for?"

I explained that I was writing a book and wanted to include some information on sex shops like this one, and that several men and two women had mentioned the Treasure Trove as being "tops in its field."

"Yes, this is a store for people who are liberated sexually. We have a very complete line of merchandise, and as you may have seen from the catalog, we will also custom-make anything a client comes up with that we don't have on hand. There are things people design that even we have never seen before."

"Could you," I said in my most distinterested journalistic manner, "perhaps tell me a little more about vibrators?"

"Of course. They're big sellers; people buy different sizes and shapes because they find different uses for them. The woman I was just waiting on wanted a thinner one than the model she had. Of course, men buy them too. For use on themselves and for their wives. They can produce fantastic sensations when used on the penis, the scrotum, or around and in the anal area. I would recommend buying one that does not make too much noise. Any complaints we've had have been from customers who say they are too loud. It's really a matter of personal taste and comes from trying different models."

"Are there any products that women buy specifically for men?"

"There are many, but one I can pinpoint is the cock ring. Cock rings are centuries old and are used to help maintain an erection and provide a sensation of increased size. They are circular rings that come in different diameters and are worn at the base of the penis and encircle the testicles as well. We have a large assortment, as you can see, in rubber, leather, and silver. Again I'd suggest to your readers that they buy one in an adjustable size so that it will fit snugly. You asked what other items women buy. They also buy French ticklers, which I guess you could say are fancy covers for cocks. They are supposed to increase the sensation for the woman. Some may give the feeling of increased penis size. Since I'm being so encyclopedic, I should warn you that even though they can provide a great feeling for women, some men say they are cheated of any sensation because of the barrier around the penis. We also recommend slipping one onto a vibrator — like a sleeve."

"What about all these other items. Who buys them?" I said, indicating a whole case and corresponding wall of rather evil-looking masks, whips, and other nether-worldly devices.

"Both men and women buy most of the merchandise in the store," he said with exquisite patience; "if something doesn't sell well, then we drop it. We're just like any other business, you know, except that we are dealing in sexual items. Whips, collars, and leather devices are bigger sellers than people might think. We're at a point in the sexual revolution where people want to explore their sexual fantasies, and we have everything they need right here. I think you'll probably get all the information you need about everything in the store from the catalog."

"Could you tell me what your best sellers are?" I asked.

"Our best seller is a T-shirt," he said.

"A T-shirt! That's something I can relate to. Which one is it?"

"That one," he said, pointing to a white T-shirt with an abstract drawing on it. "Look closer, it's not what you think it is."

And indeed it wasn't. Basically, it was a cartoon group of intertwined people indulging in an orgy.

"What's the next best seller?"

"Well, there are several things. We do a good business in bath products, body lotions, vibrators, and blow-up dolls."

"Blow-up dolls?"

"Yes, there was a big run on them during the transit strike when the mayor decreed that cars must carry at least two people. Excuse me, please, a customer is waiting," he said courteously and turned away to help her. I bought one of the catalogs and tucked it deep into a zippered compartment of my purse, thinking, If I'm run over by a truck they won't find my slip strap held up with a safety pin, they'll find *this*.

After my visit to the Treasure Trove I talked to several men and women about their shopping experiences and have come up with some conclusions based on what they told me and on my own firsthand information.

First, stores that purvey sexual equipment are like adult candy shops. The air of forbidden chocolate cherries gives these places much of their charged erotic quality. What's forbidden — and unknown — can be sexually very exciting. "I told my husband that my girl friend and I went into one of those places and he was terrifically turned on about it," said one woman I talked with. "The next week he and I went together and bought a catalog, which we look at on weekends when we have plenty of time to play in bed. We're planning to go back again and buy a couple of things."

One surprise about sex shops, at least the Treasure Trove and others that I visited, is that although they have an air of the forbidden about them, in actuality present-day dealers in erotica are usually all business. The salespeople are informed almost to the point of being clinical; they dispense information as proficiently as your neighborhood pharmacist. It's also comforting to know that they use words like "vagina," "breasts," and "cock" with the same degree of emotion that most of us have when we say "foundation makeup," "lipstick," or "mascara." No smirking or leering is involved. "We do everything we can to make the customer feel comfortable and make it easy for him or her to buy," said one of the salespeople I interviewed.

Perhaps the most interesting point about sex shops was summed up by an intelligent woman who told me, "I had made a big Christmas present of sex toys for Paul. We discovered it wasn't the gadgets but the *idea* of buying and having them that was the turn-on. In reality the sensations we make between us are far more exciting than anything the toys can provide."

A catalog is probably the best way to begin to explore the world of sex toys. Catalogs have fascinating information on the most mundane to the most esoteric sexual equipment. They are inexpensive (usually about three dollars) and provide a stimulating (or shocking) experience simply by leafing through them. You can find a variety of sex catalogs advertised in the back pages of such magazines as *Playboy* and *Playgirl*.

Basically the toys or paraphernalia found in sex shops are used to stimulate, enhance, or give reality to sexual fantasies. *All* of us have sexual fantasies. Many men and women are afraid to deal with sexual fantasies — their own or their partners' — because they think there is something unnatural or unhealthy about them. Perhaps the only unnatural or unhealthy aspect about sexual fantasy is forcing someone to become involved in something that he or she is uncomfortable with and does not wish to do. *Both* partners must be interested in the exploration of sexual fantasies, or love games, as they are sometimes called, and each partner must have complete *trust* in the other. This trust does not come about overnight. It can take many months or even years to build a deep relationship that is trusting and secure.

In addition to trust, fantasy exploration involves *imagination* and *willingness* from both partners, is basically wishful or playful, and can often bring out sides of us about which we are not consciously aware. Dominance, submissiveness, vulnerability, childishness, are but a few of the characteristics that a fantasy can reveal.

With some people, storytelling, or re-creating their fantasies verbally for their partners, is enough to give pleasure. Others want to act out their fantasies in a specific, realistic way. For playacting, preplanning is required in order to simulate "reality." Some people are intrigued by complex fantasies that involve intricate detailing and planning. They say that much of the pleasure and excitement of the fantasy lies in the preparation: in the buying of special "toys" or the wearing of special clothes, the planning of exotic "menus" or trips.

HOW TO MAKE LOVE TO A MAN

We are just beginning to have the freedom to explore deeper levels of sexual fantasy; the world of the imagination may well be the new sexual frontier.

FIFTEEN

Tricks of the Trade

Professional lovers — prostitutes, hookers, call girls, hustlers, courtesans — make sex their business, and those who are successful and stay successful have trade secrets that help keep business booming. Many of their specialties have been described throughout this book, but here are some extra-special techniques and ideas that you might find interesting as well as educational.

• "Concentration is the key to being good in bed," emphasizes a New York professional who operates out of a champagne-colored apartment with soft lighting and rare antiques on Manhattan's elegant Sutton Place. "I force myself to concentrate on what I'm doing. For instance, if I'm on top I become totally involved with the movements I'm making. If I'm doing something that he has especially requested, even though it's not something I'm crazy about, I don't let any other thought enter my brain except what my body is doing and the pleasure I'm giving. Maybe a man can't precisely tell if you're distracted or fantasizing, but I'm sure men know and feel it when you're totally and completely centered on giving them pleasure."

"Every person has something you can appreciate," says the same woman. "Even if he's not Robert Redford or Cary Grant, you can make him feel like a star if you tell him the ways he *really* is lovable. You may have to stretch your imagination, but it can be done. . . . And make sure to show a great deal of affection and care. After all, aren't most people starved for affection?"

• "Start with a bath for two," advises one attractive red-haired call girl, who points out that not only is a good soaping a sensuous experience but it "guarantees a certain degree of personal hygiene." She says she suggests a bath before getting into bed, and begins by lathering her gentleman all over, working down toward the genitals, and proceeding right to the toes. "All men want to be babied," she declares. "Then all of a sudden they get very grown-up."

• Another New York call girl learned the following trick from a New Orleans madam. Before making love she dabs some of her natural vaginal lubricant behind her ears, in the small of her back, over her breasts, and in the crook of her arm. This use of natural fragrance as a sexual attractant has a firm foundation in contemporary science. Pheromones, or substances that elicit sexual response, have been found to be present in secretions from humans, animals, and insects. Today the fragrance industry is devoting a great deal of research to these pheromones, some of which have already been incorporated into perfumes and colognes, but the natural substance in a woman's body is right there, readily available.

• "Boredom is one of the biggest sex problems men have with their wives," observes a sophisticated, highly imaginative Philadelphia pro. "The woman who puts on her face cream and wears the same nightgown night after night and does the same routine in the same room at the same time is asking for trouble. Use a little imagination and give him some variety. Have sex in the extra bedroom or the den or even on the bathroom floor. Change the lighting. Put a chair in front of a mirror and make love in it. Try out new styles in nightgowns and underwear every so often. Wear jewelry to bed — and nothing else. For some reason, men seem to love pearls. Read a sexy book to him. Wear makeup. Rub on body lotion in front of him. Put a sexy note in his jacket pocket so he'll find it when he gets to work. Change your perfume. Paint your toenails scarlet. Buy some satin sheets — the polyester ones are extra-slippery and you can get them in most discount stores."

• "The morning is the best time to make love to a man," states one professional. "Many men usually have an erection when they wake up." Science supports this view, because the male's testosterone levels, which help to dictate sexual response, are at their peak around 7:00 A.M. She goes on to say, "Morning sex is, I think, quite different from nighttime sex. It's usually more athletic and gives you a boost instead of the opposite way around. Men have told me that good sex before breakfast gives them energy all day."

• "Wear something wicked," advises a raven-haired beauty. "The big turn-on is to wear something prim and proper and add one unusual touch. Often I'll wear a black tailored suit and wear a gold pin on my lapel. If you look closely, you'll see that this elegant pin is really two people having sex. Men always have a big reaction when they discover it." Other "wicked" ideas include wearing no underpants (and letting him know), wearing a cut-out bra or cut-out sheer black underpants, a black or pink or whatever-color-pleases-him garter belt. "If you really want to surprise him," continues this lady, "wear black latex or black rubber bikini underpants, which can be purchased from catalogs or sex shops that sell erotic underwear."

• "Many women probably don't know this," says one Las Vegas professional, "but males often want to be dominated. I don't go for S & M myself,

but I sometimes suggest a game. I pretend I've tied
his hands and feet and that he must do exactly as I
command. This can be a big turn-on for a certain
type of guy."

• If a pro wants to really turn a customer on, she
will intensify his pleasure by manipulating the anus.
Usually this is done by inserting one lubricated
finger about an inch or so directly into the anus while
oral sex is taking place. "That finger must be
lubricated with saliva (and preferably a surgical jelly
or lotion) and the nail must be very short. If you are
experienced you can insert one finger even farther,
locate the prostate gland, which feels something like
a walnut, and massage this back and forth," advises
a kept woman whom I met in Los Angeles.

• But the biggest secret of the top-quality
professional remains *focus* and *undiluted, undivided*
attention to the man she's in bed with. "I focus totally
and completely on the man. I try and make him feel
he's the only man in the world, that he's the sexiest,
most desirable, most wonderful lover I could
possibly have," said one articulate call girl who is
paid over one thousand dollars a night for her
services by an international clientele.

"Nothing is a bigger turn-on "she said,"than
knowing you are the object of someone's desire and
that *you* are the sole focus of love and attention.
Surely the best way to make love to a man is to let
him know that you are truly carried away by desire."

SIXTEEN

The Story of J.

Even though she was on a split-second timetable, Joanna took a few extra minutes to straighten up the papers on her desk and place them in three piles. "Those of us who are condemned to neatness . . ." she muttered to herself as she tapped the corners of the unruly papers into tidy right angles.

A few minutes late now, she hurried out of the office into the cool November evening. She headed uptown to a special French bakery, thinking, as she stepped up her pace, of what she would wear to the cocktail party she was going to that evening. In the shop the fragrance of freshly cooked cakes and babas au rhum was so overpowering that she had to exert utmost control to restrain herself from buying her favorite buttery almond tart and eating it right there on the spot. Instead, she coolly picked up half a pound of delicate meringue cookies (27 calories each, she remembered from her calorie counter), and continued to her next destination.

"Four breasts and two legs," she told the woman.

"Right, honey, and you want them extra-crispy, don't you?"

Joanna nodded yes, and tucked the red-and-white-striped Kentucky Fried Chicken bag under her arm. She reached home barely ten minutes off schedule.

It was six-fifteen and she was to meet Michael at the Crawford cocktail party at seven-thirty. But before then she had plenty to do.

She checked the freezer to see how its contents were coming along. She uncorked the special bottle of Chianti, hid it under the cupboard with the little packet from the florist, took out a wicker basket, lined it with a red-and-white-checked cloth, hid this under the sink, and located twelve small candles, which she placed in demitasse saucers on the far side of each step of the staircase leading to the bedroom.

The bed had been freshly made that morning. She put out two more flowered sheets on the dresser and tucked something square under the pillow. The phone rang.

"Hello? . . . Hi, Frank. . . . Yes, I had just called you to confirm the time. We should be home by eight-thirty. If you get here by quarter of nine, we should be in perfect shape. Just ring. I'll leave a check for you in your jacket pocket. See you later."

She showered hastily, cleaned the tub, tidied up the towels, and gave a finishing flourish of Comet to the sink so that it sparkled. She sprayed some Chanel

No. 19 on herself and, extravagantly, sprayed some more on the towels. She took some extra care with her makeup and hair, slipped into a burgundy-colored silk dress, some sexy strappy high-heeled shoes, and gave herself a critical look in the mirror. Not too bad, she thought, feeling good about the disciplinary measures she'd taken in the pastry shop. She turned to put on her coat, hesitated, walked back to the bedroom, took off her pantyhose, and replaced them with a fragile white satin garter belt and stockings that had thin black seams running up the back.

She reached the Crawfords' at seven-thirty sharp and found Michael already there.

"Hello, my love," he said, giving her a kiss. "You look lovely tonight, particularly your legs." He grinned at her.

"My mother told me the secret to being sexy had something to do with stockings, but she never explained further. I'm glad you noticed. I thought that once we started living together your eyes would begin to lose their elasticity."

"Never," he promised solemnly. "Let's go and talk to our pals; otherwise people might think we're in love. By the way, should we ask Norman and Alexandra if they want to have a bite to eat with us after this is over?"

"I've got a tough day at work tomorrow and I'd really rather we go on home, if you don't mind. We can just fix a quick sandwich."

"Fine with me."

By eight-twenty they'd said their good-byes and were heading the six blocks home to their apartment.

"Oh, Michael, we need some milk for breakfast, do you mind stopping for it? I'm going to run home; I've got to go to the bathroom, *badly!*"

"Sure. I'll be along in a minute."

As soon as Michael headed in the other direction, Joanna speeded up to a run, dashed into the house to get a match, and lit each candle along the staircase. She went into the bedroom, took off everything except her garter belt and stockings, and wrapped a silk kimono around her. When Michael came in the door she was standing at the top of the stairs.

"What's happening? There was a fire sale on candles?" he asked, trying to deadpan, but a smile got the better of him.

"I'm going to light *your* fire," said Joanna with a demure, innocent look on her face. "Why don't you 'slip into something comfortable' and we can have another drink if you like."

While Michael was upstairs, the doorbell rang. Joanna ushered Frank in and told him, "He's changing, stay here in the hall, and when he comes downstairs just go right into the bedroom and set up."

"Who was that?" asked Michael, coming down into the living room.

"Oh, just some kid who rang the doorbell by mistake. Come, let's sit, and then I'll make a sandwich for us."

"Now, Joanna, what's going on —"

"If you wait patiently for four minutes, you'll find out."

"Find out what?"

"How I intend to seduce you."

"It's about time!"

In a few minutes Joanna took Michael by the hand and led him into the bedroom, where Frank had set up a table draped with flowered sheets.

"This is Frank Bosco, he's going to give you a massage," Joanna told an astonished Michael, as she stretched out on the bed nearby.

"I'm sure I've died and gone to heaven," said Michael to Joanna when Frank had left. "A massage in our own house. That's one of the nicest things anyone has ever done for me."

"Well, it's not over yet. Why don't you settle yourself among the pillows and see what happens next."

Joanna disappeared into the kitchen and came out with the wicker picnic basket in one hand and a bottle of wine, which had a tiny bunch of fresh daisies tied to it, in the other. Inside the basket was a crusty loaf of bread, six extra-crispy pieces of fried chicken, iced carrot and celery slices, two huge napkins, and two crystal goblets. She spread the tablecloth over the comforter.

"Your favorite dinner is served," announced Joanna, putting on a Frank Sinatra album, another

special favorite of theirs. "I think you should also
know I love you very much!"

Much laughing, much merriment, much kissing,
and much eating for the next hour, interrupted only
by Joanna's trip to the kitchen for the dessert. Four
servings of a low-cal but delectable homemade lemon
ice and ten little meringue cookies later, Joanna
slowly and deliberately put away their picnic things,
clicked off the stereo, and lit a candle. Slipping out of
her kimono, leaving it in a lovely heap on the floor,
she drew Michael up by the hand and turned back
the scented bedcovers and fresh sheets, motioning to
him to tuck in next to her. She reached under the
pillow for a thick book, which had been earmarked
on certain pages. Opening the book she began
reading, slowly, in a soft voice.

*"As you know dearest, I never use obscene phrases
in speaking. You have never heard me, have you,
utter an unfit word before others. When men tell in
my presence their filthy or lecherous stories I hardly
smile. Yet you seem to turn me into a beast. It was
you yourself you naughty shameless girl who first
led the way. It was not I who first touched you long
ago down at Ringsend. It was you who slid your
hand down inside my trousers and –"*

"*Who* is this woman?" asked Michael.

*"– pulled my shirt softly aside and touched my prick
with your long tickling fingers and gradually took it
all. . . . It was your lips too which first uttered an
obscene word. I remember well that night in bed in*

142

Pola. Tired of lying under a man one night you tore
off your chemise violently and got on top of me to
ride me naked. You stuck my prick into your cunt
and began to ride me up and down –"

"There's a smart woman," Michael interrupted.

"You say when I go back, [Joanna continued, even
more slowly, not answering] *you will suck me off*
and you want me to lick your cunt, you depraved
blackguard. I hope you will surprise me sometime
when I'm asleep dressed, steal over to me with a
whore's glow in your slumbrous eyes, gently undo
button after button in the fly of my trousers and
gently take your lover's fat mickey, lap it up in your
moist mouth and suck away at it till it gets fatter and
stiffer and comes off in your mouth. . . ."

"Who are these people? What wonderful wicked
things they do with each other! Joanna —"

"If you must know," said Joanna, closing the
book, "it's one of the most famous writers in the
English language, writing to the woman he's deeply
in love with. He was in Italy and she was in Ireland.
The year was 1909. The book is James Joyce's *Letters*.
But," Joanna said, kissing him in the ear and
reaching up to turn off the reading light, "one touch
is worth a thousand letters, as Nora so well knew." A
single candle flickered, casting dancing shadows on
the ceiling.

"Now," said Joanna to Michael, "I'm about to
make love to you."